Handbook of Urological Endoscopy

Handbook of Urological Endoscopy

J. G. Gow
M.D., Ch.M., F.R.C.S.
Consultant Urologist,
Mossley Hill Hospital, Liverpool

H. H. Hopkins
F.R.S.
Professor of Optics,
University of Reading

With contributions by

D. M. Wallace
O.B.E., B.Sc., M.S., F.R.C.S.
Professor of Urology,
University of Riyadh,
Saudi Arabia

and

A. G. England

B.Sc., M.B., Ch.B.
Regional Scientific Officer,
Mersey Regional Health Authority,
Liverpool

CHURCHILL LIVINGSTONE
EDINBURGH LONDON AND NEW YORK 1978

CHURCHILL LIVINGSTONE
Medical Division of Longman Group Limited

Distributed in the United States of America by
Longman Inc., 19 West 44th Street, New York,
N.Y. 10036 and by associated companies,
branches and representatives throughout
the world.

First published 1978

ISBN 0 443 01419 1   .

British Library Cataloguing in Publication Data
Gow, J G
    Handbook of urological endoscopy.
    1. Urinary organs—Diseases—Diagnosis
    2. Endoscope and endoscopy
    I. Title   II. Hopkins, H H
    616.6   RC901.7.E/   77-30315

Printed in Great Britain by T. & A. Constable, Edinburgh

Preface

Recent development in optics and in the design of optical systems and light sources have now advanced the practice of urological endoscopy to a state where it can fulfil a primary role in diagnostic urology. The success of urological practice depends on the surgeon's investigative power as well as his clinical acumen. Modern endoscopy provides this basis of clear and accurate clinical information.

This book is, therefore, addressed to young urologists who are embarking on a career in this discipline, and who will find that a high proportion of their work involves endoscopy. It is not intended as a comprehensive account of all urological conditions, but does attempt to demonstrate the common lesions most frequently encountered in urological practice as well as the importance of endoscopy in their appraisal.

The book should also be of value to general surgeons with an interest in urology, a group that is likely to continue in the United Kingdom until more specialised units are formed.

The first chapter on the history of urology has been written by Mr David Wallace, and we are most grateful to him for such an outstanding introduction. We are also grateful to Dr Gordon England for his chapter describing a new technique for the production of sterile pyrogen-free water for use in endoscopic procedures. After Mr Wallace's introduction, the next six chapters are devoted to descriptions of the technical aspects of urological endoscopy. The remainder of the book takes the form of a colour atlas of endoscopic photographs of various urological conditions with brief textual descriptions. We have kept the text to a minimum and have omitted all but the most important references.

It is to be hoped that this book will reflect in some small way the concern and enthusiasm engendered by the harmonious co-operation of the two authors engaged for nearly twenty years in furthering the development of techniques in which there has been mutual fascination and interest.

1978   J.G.G
                                                        H.H.H

Acknowledgements

The two authors have long believed that the advances made in modern optical techniques, both in their application to medicine and photography, would be of value to trainee urologists. It was this belief which inspired them to produce this volume.

In such a volume many people have been involved. First we must express appreciation to the anaesthetists, Dr Mackinnon, Dr Ryan and Dr Jarvie for long hours of patient forebearance. We are also grateful to Dr Gibson for his helpful advice on the sterilisation of endoscopic instruments and for allowing us to publish some of his data. Dr Dobbie has been most considerate in advising us of problems concerning surgical diathermy and to him we are most grateful. We are especially indebted to Dr Pugh for providing the excellent microphotographs of tumours to put alongside the cystoscopic photographs.

The excellence and precision of the photographs would not have been achieved without the help and encouragement of Mr S. Dobson, The Department of Physics, Reading University, and to him we owe a special debt of gratitude.

This manuscript could not have been prepared without the uncomplaining assistance of Mrs Barbara Worthington, who has typed and re-typed many of the chapters with cheerful enthusiasm, and who has worked hours long beyond the call of duty.

Contents

1. History of cystoscopy

Professor D. M. Wallace, O.B.E., B.Sc., M.S., F.R.C.S.

Even before the days of the Romans, man's natural curiosity concerning the functions of the human body, led him to produce a variety of instruments, some of which resemble the diagnostic equipment of today. It is assumed that these, rather crude, instruments were designed for the inspection of the vagina or rectum.

It is however, only in the last century that technical advances have allowed the development of more complex diagnostic methods. It is not generally realised that up to the beginning of the last century, sunlight, animal fat or vegetable oils, were the only sources of light available. The stimulus to endoscopy came with the development of better light sources, at first, mineral oil with additions to make the flame brighter, then the electric filament lamp, especially the Mignon version, and even more recently, the fibre optic non-coherent light cables.

Some of these technical developments were adopted into clinical practice with extreme speed, others took longer.

Bozzini's lichtleiter

It was not until 1806 that any attempt was made to visualise body cavities. In this year Bozzini demonstrated his new invention to the Academy of Medicine in Vienna, in the Hosephinian Library of the then Academy (now the Institut für die Geschichte der Medizin der Universität, Wien), but received scant encouragement. His original instrument, which is now preserved in the American College of Surgeons, Chicago, was clumsy and ineffective, but it did represent the first serious attempt to inspect body cavities (Fig. 1.1). It was an instrument designed for a multitude of functions; it could be fitted with a speculum, with an angled mirror at the end, which was probably designed for inspection of the nasopharynx. Another instrument, with several attachments, few of them bladed and one with a urethral speculum, was made for examination of the anal canal, the rectum and the vagina.

The urethral speculum, made of silver, was an open-ended tube and must have been used with air insufflation. It could, only under extreme difficulty, have been used in an air-filled bladder. The area of the urethral or bladder wall available for inspection, could have

been only a few millimetres in diameter.

The main instrument is made of silver, covered in shark skin to prevent burns. Within the instrument a beeswax candle, spring loaded, provided a light, the flame of which was in a constant position. To one side of the light, and shielded from the light by a mirror, was the observation eyepiece in line with the axis of the examining speculum.

The whole instrument had to be kept vertical and presumably the patient was positioned around the instrument.

The two major causes of the lichtleiter's failure to be adopted as an endoscopic method, were the absence of optical magnification and a poor and uncontrollable light source.

The mid 19th century

Several attempts at endoscopy were made by a variety of clinicians, but it was not until Désormeaux of Paris produced his endoscope, that endoscopy became a

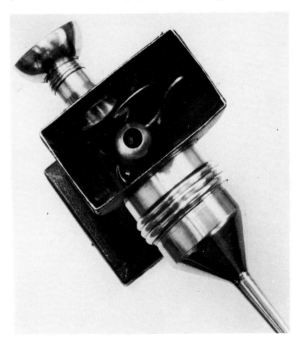

Fig. 1.1 Bozzini's lichtleiter 1806.
View from above to show mirror inspection eyepiece and spring loaded candle.

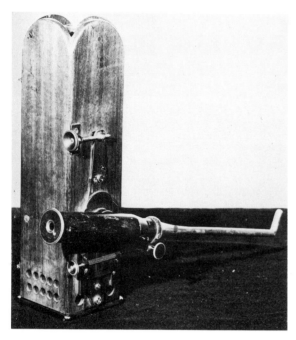

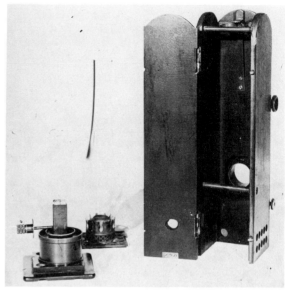

Figs. 1.2 and 1.3   Cruise instrument (2 views).

practical, though difficult method of investigation. Désormeaux, the father of endoscopy, designed his instrument around a paraffin flame, which was made to burn more brightly by the addition of turpentine. The metal lamp-housing tended to become very hot and there is at least one comment in the contemporary reports about burns to the surgeon's face. Attached to the lamp-housing was the endoscope proper. The light was reflected down the endoscope by means of an angled mirror, perforated to allow inspection along the endoscope axis. A variety of fittings were available including an optical method of magnification attached at the external end.

Cruise of Dublin was a friend and a close collaborator of Désormeaux. Cruise's instrument (Figs. 1.2. & 1.3) preserved in the Royal College of Surgeons in Dublin, is similar to that of Désormeaux, but because of the risk of burns this instrument is housed in a wooden box. Cruise used the flame edge on to the reflecting mirror, and increased its brilliance by adding camphor. The fittings however, are even more interesting, especially the urethral cannula. This cannula, one of which is open-ended, would have been used in an air-filled bladder, but Fenwick describes a cannula devised by Cruise which was fitted with a lateral window, and an angled proximal mirror. Fenwick reports that, when the lateral window was set in the axis of the tube, light was reflected back, which made observation of the lateral wall of the bladder difficult, but this could be prevented by setting the window at a slight angle. There is no doubt, that these men, through a bladder cavity filled with boracic solution, were able to inspect the greater part of the bladder mucosa.

The technique and the physical contortions on the part of both patient and surgeon resulted in this method failing to be generally adopted. However, at this time, electricity was being developed as an alternative source of light.

The late 19th century

Brueck, a dentist of Breslau, was experimenting with a platinum filament lamp heated to a white heat as a source of light. His earliest effort, a dental mirror, was cooled by a stream of water circulating behind the filament. Subsequently, he developed his interests to include the bladder. Here he inserted one of his glass tubes with a cooling jacket (Figs 1.4 & 1.5) into the rectum, and by passing a straight speculum into the bladder was able to see a small portion of the bladder wall by the light transmitted from the lamp in the rectum. This instrument is also preserved in Wien.

A colleague of Brueck, a gynaecologist called Schramm, of Dresden, attempted the same procedure and claimed that with Brueck's lamp in the vagina he could 'in a thin woman in a darkened room' make out the shape of the uterus and ovaries.

Neither of these techniques were of any significance, but the knowledge of their efforts spread to Berlin, where a young urologist decided to re-open the whole question of endoscopy. Max Nitze had two fundamental ideas: firstly to use lenses in the form of a miniature telescope to magnify the image down the endoscope, and secondly to illuminate the interior of the bladder by a water-cooled electric platinum filament lamp. His first efforts to

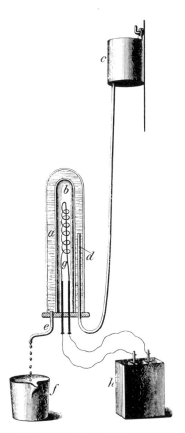

Fig. 1.4   Diagram of Brueck's irrigating system.

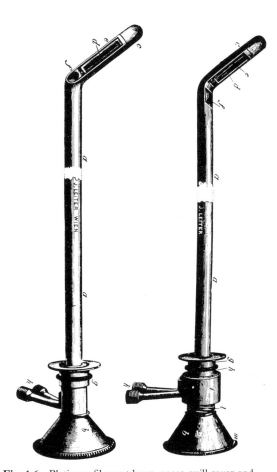

Fig. 1.6   Platinum filament lamp, goose quill cover and irrigating system 1878.

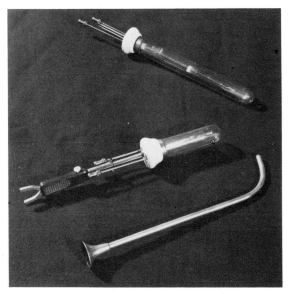

Fig. 1.5   Lamps for vaginal and rectal insertion with a direct vision non-optical cannula for inspection of the posterior bladder wall.

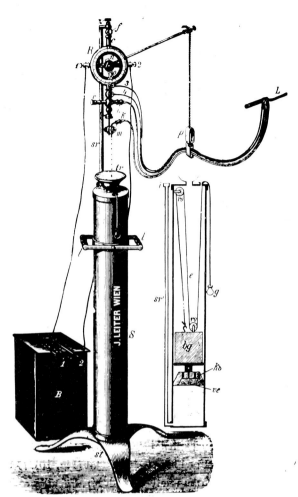

Fig. 1.7   Irrigating system to keep lamp cool.

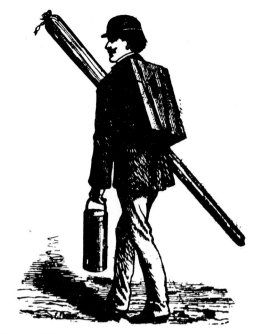

Fig. 1.8   Well equipped urologist proceeding to a cystoscopy.

produce a satisfactory instrument in Berlin were in-complete, so he moved to the clinic of Von Dittel in Vienna. Here, he was allowed every opportunity to develop his technique, and at the same time he colla-borated with a senior surgical instrument maker, Leiter, and a lamp maker, Heyman.

Their first instrument was cumbersome (Fig. 1.6). The filament was a platinum spiral inside a goose quill; it was kept cool by a complicated irrigation system (Fig. 1.7) and the telescope design was far from perfect. The urologist of those days required a porter to carry his cumbersome and somewhat temperamental equipment (Fig. 1.8). Sir Henry Thompson of St. Peter's Hospital, wrote scathingly of this instrument and saw no future in it. Unfortunately, even though Sir Henry possessed a replica of this instrument, it has since been lost.

The Mignon lamp

Heat from the white hot platinum filament was the

limiting factor in cystoscopy, but in England and America almost simultaneously, a major technical advance occurred. Swan, in 1878, demonstrated in Newcastle, that a lamp could be produced which, in vacuum, was neither too hot nor liable to burn out. Edison, a few months later, using a carbon filament in a vacuum, produced a similar lamp. This event, the discovery of a vacuum lamp, rapidly resulted in the production of the Mignon lamp, a small vacuum lamp which could be inserted at the end of a cystoscope into a water-filled bladder. This lamp was reliable and unlikely to damage, by heat, the patient's bladder wall (Fig. 1.9).

The three main Nitze-type cystoscopes are (Fig. 1.10)

1. The urethroscope, developed in Berlin with the goose quill lamp and irrigating system (1876)
2. The urethroscope/cystoscope, improved optically by Leiter but still with a complicated irrigating system (1878)
3. The Nitze-Leiter cystoscope of 1880, fitted with the improved telescope and the Mignon vacuum lamp without an irrigating system.

The next few years are interesting because Von Dittel gave Nitze all the credit for the development of this instrument. Leiter and Nitze were to write a book on the technical and clinical aspects of urology, but the Vienna of those days, to a handsome young man, must have offered considerable distractions. The co-authorship book failed to materialise, the collaboration broke up and Nitze returned to Berlin, where he and

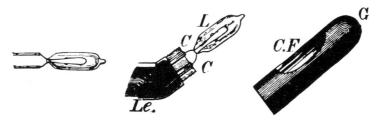

Fig. 1.9 Mignon lamp 1880.

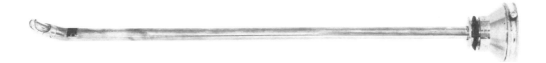

Fig. 1.10 One of the earliest Nitze Leiter cystoscopes fitted with the Mignon lamp.

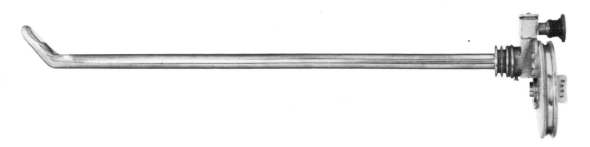

Figs. 1.11 and 1.12 Nitze photographic cystoscope (2 views).

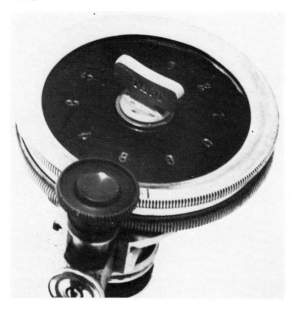

his University department continued to produce, and modify, improvements in cystoscopes.

The number of cystoscopes which evolved over the next twenty years is incredible, but one modification is worthy of a more detailed description. The Amici prism marks a different era. The original cystoscope had either a direct forward-looking visual axis or the axis was altered through 90° by means of a terminal right-angled prism. This prism had one defect, in that it produced an inverted image, a mirror image. The Amici prism (a roofprism) was developed for use in cystoscopes in 1906. In brief, an extra prism was cut in the first prism on the hypotenuse face so that the image underwent a double reflection and thus became optically corrected. This prism is an essential component of all European instruments, but the American instruments of those days were corrected by the insertion of an additional prism in the shaft of the cystoscope.

The various modifications to the classical Nitze instrument mainly stemmed from Nitze's close collaboration with Herschman and Hartweg, instrument makers of Berlin. A photographic cystoscope allowed Kutner to take photographs inside the bladder in 1890 (Figs. 1.11 & 1.12). A diathermy cystoscope, credited to

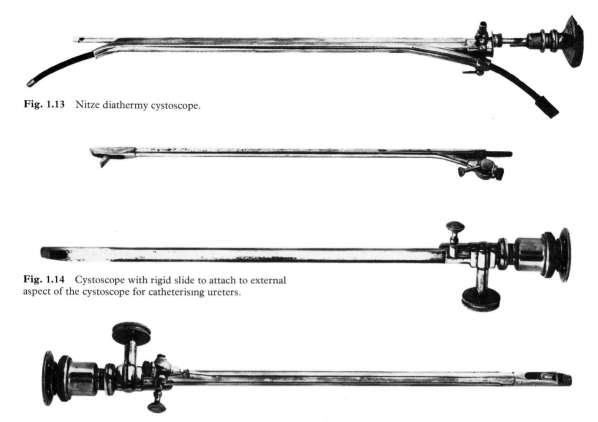

Fig. 1.13   Nitze diathermy cystoscope.

Fig. 1.14   Cystoscope with rigid slide to attach to external
aspect of the cystoscope for catheterising ureters.

Fig. 1.15   Slide attached to outside of sheath with movable lever.

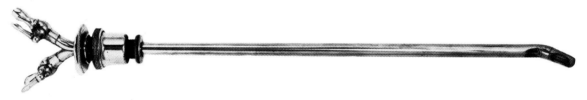

Fig. 1.16   Guterback's irrigating system for use prior to inserting telescope.

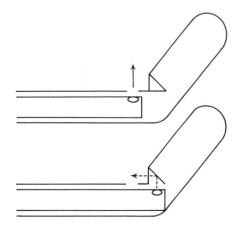

Fig. 1.17   Method of increasing the optical range by the use of prisms.

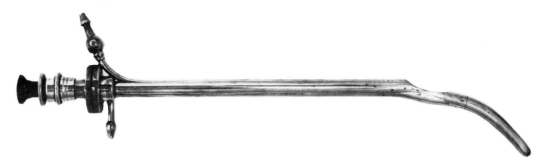

Fig. 1.18 Woddislo instrument with unique curve to scope and with the lamp built into the spine of the sheath.

Nitze, where a large electrode could be passed was the forerunner of the Kidds diathermy instrument (Fig. 1.13). Several cystoscopes were produced with an interchangeable external slide to allow catheterisation (Figs. 1.14 & 1.15).

Albarran in 1896, produced a cystoscope with an internal lever working inside the sheath to facilitate ureteric catheterisation. Brenner produced an instrument with a direct vision telescope and a fixed internal catheterising channel. Guterback used a double luman cannula for irrigation of the bladder prior to inspection (Fig. 1.16), but none of these represented a major optical advance.

Two attempts were made to increase the optical range by the addition of prisms. In the first, a prism fixed below the lamp (Fig. 1.17) could be brought into use by advancing the telescope, while a second model allowed a prism to be rotated over the end of the telescope. In both of these models the image, because of the double mirror effect, was both reversed and inverted.

Wossidlo, a urologist from Saxony spent part of his professional life in South Africa before returning to Berlin. He evolved a cystoscope with a completely different shape and with the lamp inserted in the spire of the sheath, a device which was later copied by some of the prostatic punch manufacturers (Fig. 1.18).

The British experience
In Britain the endoscope had failed to make any significant impact, although Newman of Glasgow had invented an instrument and he was certainly the first to catheterise the female ureters (1886) in Britain (Fig. 1.19). Unfortunately this instrument has also been lost, but was a forerunner of both Luys and the Kelly open tube type of cystoscope.

This Scottish invention passed unnoticed by the urologists south of the border, who began to rely on cystoscopes made in Berlin.

It was not until 1916 that the source of cystoscopes and means of repairing cystoscopes became a national problem. In this year, the Government commissioned

Weiss, an old established instrument maker with a long-standing interest in urology (Weiss collection of lithotrites in Institute of Urology, London), to develop a British cystoscope. A small unit of three men began to develop a copy of what was then the popular cystoscope designed by Ringleb, but shortly afterwards, the development unit left Weiss to become the Genitourinary Manufacturing Company. From this simple wartime necessity, numerous offshoots of other companies have developed. British urology however, is a very personal speciality, so that a host of modifications, different types, different fittings and complete lack of standardisation became the pattern in the interwar years.

The advent of 1939–45 and the large numbers of Brown-Buerger cystoscopes left in Europe at the end of hostilities finally convinced British urologists that some form of standardisation was essential, not only for urology in Britain, but also in the interests of world trade.

The most recent, and perhaps, the most significant contribution to urology from Britain came with the closer collaboration between urology and physics, as practised by Professor Hopkins.

Although fibre-optics had been described as a method of conducting light around corners by Professor Hopkins in 1954, it took several years before this form of illumination was adopted by the cystoscope manufacturers and even longer before his second contribution, solid rod lenses, was also incorporated as a standard form of cystoscopic observation.

The American experience
The observation of the bladder in America was made popular by gynaecologists, such as Kelly who, using short open-ended tubes with the patient in the knee-chest position or reversed Trendelenburg, were able to conduct a limited inspection of the bladder wall. This tradition has been handed down to the American urologists in the form of the Braasch cystoscope, and the many modifications of the punch resectoscope.

It was Otis who, following a visit to Berlin, first introduced the Nitze-type instrument to America.

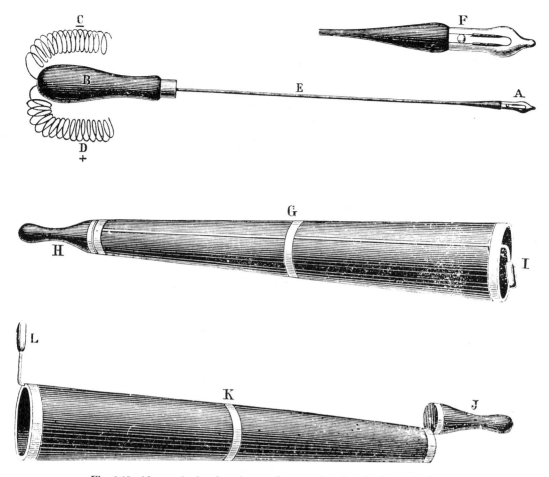

Fig. 1.19 Newman's electric endoscope for ureteric catheterisation in the female.

Tilden Brown and Leo Buerger were able to persuade Wappler, the founder of the most famous firm of cytoscope makers, to develop an American cystoscope, which for the last seventy years, has remained virtually unchanged as the pre-eminent cystoscope. It is now recognised and used worldwide. For any instrument to have been in regular use for so long speaks highly for its design and the principle of interchangeability and standardisation of components. The advent of new technology will allow the dearly loved classical Brown-Buerger cystoscope to retire with both dignity and honour.

REFERENCES

Places where cystoscopes are preserved

History Museum, University of Leiden.
History Museum, University of Vienna.
Royal College of Surgeons, Dublin.
American College of Surgeons, Chicago.
University of Caracas, Venezuala.
École de Médicin, Paris.
Institute of Urology, University of London.
Department of Urological History, Cook County Hospital, Chicago.
Institute for History of Medicine, Berlin.

Dates

Bozzino (Philip) 1773–1809
Leopold von Dittel 1815–1898
Joseph Leiter 1830–1892
Max Nitze 1848–1904
Désormeaux, A. J. 1815–1882
Francis Cruise
Leopold Casper
Alex Brenner

Two books

Fenwick, E. Harry. *Handbook of Clinical Electric Light Cystoscope*, 1904.
Newman. *Lectures to Practitioners on Surgical Diseases of the Kidney*, 1888.

2. The endoscope

The evolution of the cystoscope has been fully discussed in Chapter 1. Gone are the days when the endoscopist depended on an instrument illuminated at its tip by a small lamp of inadequate power and doubtful reliability. Now a more sophisticated system based on an external high intensity light source fed to the instrument through a fibre cable and transmitted through the telescope by a fibre light bundle, so arranged, to illuminate the area subtended by the objective lens, is standard practice. It is essential that the modern endoscopist should consider cystourethroscopy not as an isolated investigation, but part of a more sophisticated system embracing most situations associated with this examination. It should, therefore, be possible to undertake ureteric catheterisation, biopsy of suspected areas, resection of tumour or prostate and removal of small foreign bodies without removing the sheath used for the initial examination. For such a system to be successful, continuous irrigation must be available, as no satisfactory cystourethroscopy can be carried out without such facilities. The one exception is cystoscopic litholapaxy, as the sheath is an integral part of the mechanism and cannot be separated.

The examining sheath

The examining instrument consists of a hollow tube, constructed from stainless steel, with a small angle at the tip. Prior to the introduction of the instrument, an obturator is inserted to prevent trauma, especially to the external meatus. Figure 2.1 shows three instruments of different dimensions, size 17.5, 22 and 24 charrière. These are colour-coded to help identification. Occasionally urethral lesions require diathermy treatment and this is best carried out through a panendoscope sheath which is similar to the examining sheath but which does not have a terminal beak. Figure 2.2 shows 3 sheaths, size 18, 22 and 24, with the same colour-coding as the examining sheaths.

The instruments shown are fitted with British Standard irrigation connections but these are being

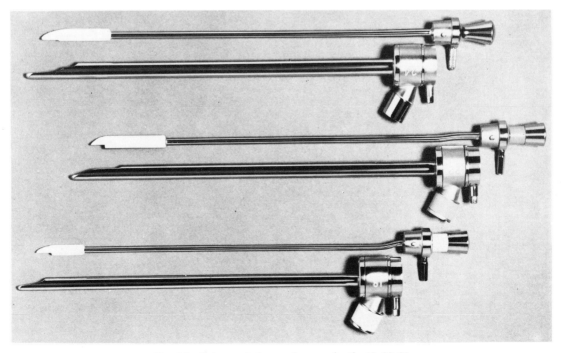

Fig. 2.2 Colour coded panendoscope sheaths 18, 22, 24.

replaced by Luer fittings to conform with the agreed standard for the European Community. These sheaths cannot be used for diathermy resection and are being employed less and less in view of the concept of a rationalised integrated system.

The resectoscope sheath

The resectoscope sheath is an insulated tube constructed from woven glass fibre bonded with an epoxy resin, which is wound round a mandrel, until the desired thickness is obtained. This one has become the sheath of choice. The dark colour is obtained by introducing the pigment during the winding process. Such tubes have been tested and failure only occurred, when it was exposed to a load far in excess of that likely to be experienced in normal use. Figure 2.3 shows three sheaths of different dimensions, size 24, 26 and 28 charriére, again colour-coded to facilitate recognition. As these sheaths have a straight beak at the end, which can be either short or long, it is advisable, to avoid posterior urethral trauma, to use a spring loaded articulated obturator (Fig. 2.4), which forms an angle at the tip when it is pressed fully home into the sheath. Some continental manufacturers construct the main shaft of the sheath in metal, bonding an insulated material on the tip. This has the advantage of a greater strength as fracture of the shaft of the bonded glass fibre material has been reported. But its disadvantage is a weakness at the tip where the insulated material is attached to the metal. Operators have experienced a fracture at this point. This can be an embarrassment, as it can be difficult to remove through the urethra. These sheaths are made in sizes 24, 26 and 28 charriére. The size 26 is the normal size for routine use, but the ultimate criteria is the size of the patient's urethra and size 28 should only be used on rare occasions when the urethra is wide, as in these cases, there is additional risk of urethral or meatal stricture. The irrigation system is attached to the side of the sheath and the types of fluid are discussed in a later chapter.

The telescope

A typical modern telescope is the System 80, which is, at present, available in three angles, 0°, 30° and 70° (Fig. 2.5). The 0° is direct vision, 30° forward oblique, 70° lateral (Fig. 2.6). All have a field of view, under

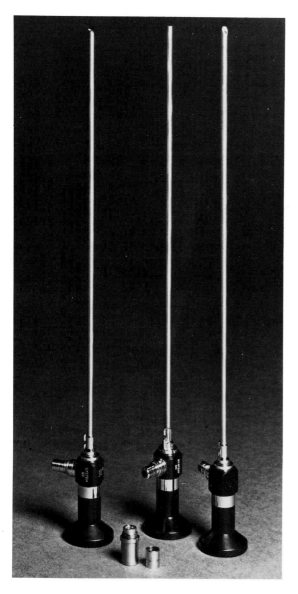

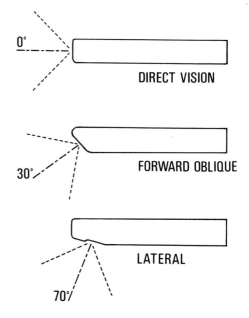

Figs. 2.5 and 2.6   Three telescopes 0°, 30° and 70° with adaptors for different fibre light cables.

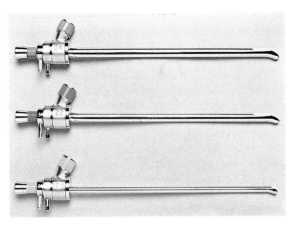

Fig. 2.1
Colour coded examining sheaths 17·5, 22, 24.

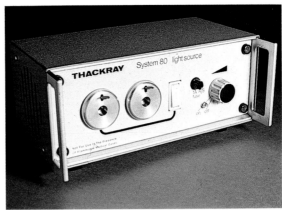

Fig. 2.7
High intensity external light source.

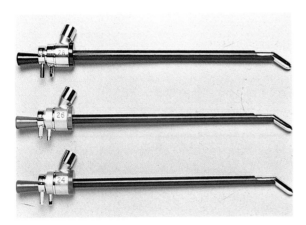

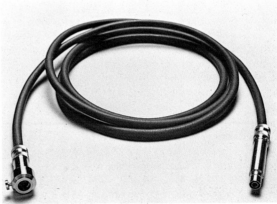

Fig. 2.8
Fibre light cable.

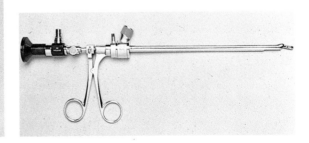

Figs. 2.3 and 2.4
Colour coded Resectoscope sheaths with
articulated beak 24, 26, 28.

Fig. 2.10
Biopsy forceps (black and white).

water, of 70°, and all use optical glass-fibres for illumination. Each telescope is supplied complete with two screw-on adapters, which facilitate the use of alternative makes of fibre-light guides. Fibre-light guides connect with British Standard, Wolf or Storz fittings, and can all be used with System 80 telescopes, by varying the appropriate adapter, which should be screwed to the telescope as described above. System 80 telescopes are designed to be used in conjunction with System 80 instruments. They can also be fitted to instruments made by other manufacturers, provided there is suitable modification or adaption. Inserting a System 80 telescope into a sheath always needs an interconnecting bridge. This can be a simple extension piece, a panendoscope bridge, a resectoscope mechanism or a catheterising attachment. All the telescopes will fit any of the bridges mentioned.

The light source

The light is provided by a high intensity light source. Figure 2.7 is a typical example. The particular light source contains two Quartz Halogen projection lamps easily changeable, one to be kept in reserve, in case of failure. Both are cooled by an axial fan. The intensity is controlled by a solid state resistance. To protect the life of these lamps the illumination should be increased slowly from 0 to the required brightness.

Light cable

The light is conveyed to the telescope by a fibre light cable, (Fig. 2.8). To obtain the maximum efficient transmission of light the terminal of the cable, which attaches it to the telescope, should be compatible and specially made to fit accurately with the bundle in the telescope,

as any undue separation at the point of contact or any difference in the diameter of the telescope fibre bundle and the light guide will result in light loss. As much as 20 per cent can be lost at each interface if the contact is inaccurate. Another important factor is the relationship between flexibility and strength. Extremely flexible guides are, unquestionably, easier to use and all other factors being equal, would be the first choice. However, flexible guides are more fragile, and consequently, more prone to damage. As they are costly, a happy medium has to be struck between flexibility and fragility. The rigid guide, undoubtedly, gives many times the length of service and it is only a question of time for the user to become accustomed to its greater rigidity and readily adapt to the diminished flexibility. As a result this guide is beginning to replace the more flexible unit. All cables conform to the British Standard Specification. They should be capable of repeated flexion around a mandrel of not more than 80 mm in diameter, without damage, should be approximately 1·8 metres in length and should be covered by a protective covering, in the case of the one illustrated, stainless steel.

These are the basic instrumental requirements of an initial cystourethroscopy examination; but the modern system must be able to do much more.

Ureteric catheterisation

This is an examination which is being carried out less and less frequently due to the improvement in X-ray techniques of the renal tract using a high dose injection technique which, in most cases, gives a very accurate picture of the pelvicalyceal system. Nevertheless, it may be required, when a precise diagnosis cannot be unequivocally made or when it is important to investigate

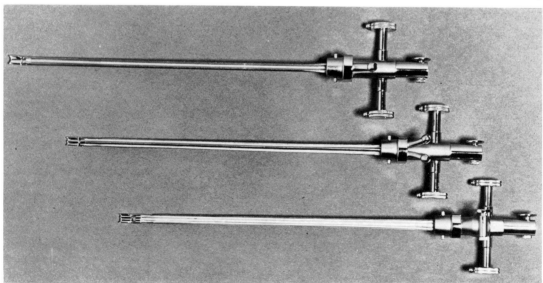

Fig. 2.9 Catheter deflector with albarran bar.

segregated specimens of urine. For this investigation, a catheter deflector incorporating an albarran bar is used (Fig. 2.9). This can have either a simple or double catheterising attachment with or without taps. Without taps is preferable as they are unnecessary, tend to constrict the lumen and are a nuisance to the operator. If segregated specimens are required either a Braasch bulb or chevassu catheter is used and for this the single attachment is essential. Either the 30° or 70° telescope can be used, depending on the anatomical situation of the ureteric orifice.

Tissue biopsy

The method employed depends on the technique of individual operators and is carried out either by biopsy forceps (Fig. 2.10), or diathermy excision by the resectoscope. Many pathologists prefer specimens produced by the biopsy forceps as they find precise diagnosis and especially the staging of tumours at the edges difficult, following diathermy excision because of necrosis and considerable damage to peripheral cells. The instrument is passed through a 24 or 26 charriére sheath and a 30° telescope is used. With this telescope, it is difficult to obtain specimens from some areas of the bladder, especially the roof proximal to the bladder neck, but suprapubic abdominal pressure will often bring such a lesion within the range of the instrument.

Transurethral resection of the prostate and tumour

Today there are numerous resectoscopes, all made to the various idiosyncrasies of different urologists. Figure 2.11 shows four examples, the Nesbit, the Schranz, the Iglesias and the Mitchell. There are, however, many more and all have their advocates. It is essential, for the beginner to become acquainted with one particular instrument and to stick to it until he learns the rudiments of his art. Once he has mastered the technique, transferring from one to another takes little time, and he can then adjust to the one that he feels is most suitable to this method. Once having decided, he would do well to keep to the one, which has become a trusted friend. Figure 2.12 shows the loops and a diathermy electrode that are used for resection and coagulation, colour-coded for size, a flat diathermy electrode, which is very useful for controlling haemorrhage at the bladder neck and also for coagulating areas at the periphery of tumours. Also shown is a roller type electrode, which is an asset for controlling haemorrhage at the end of a prostatic resection.

Litholapaxy

Provided the calculi are less than 2 cms in diameter the cystoscopic lithotrite manufactured by Storz (Fig. 2.13), enables the operator to undertake a rapid and effective

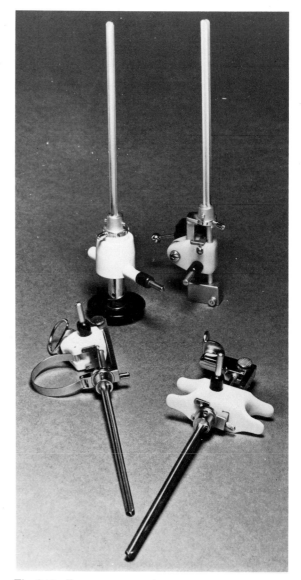

Fig. 2.11 Four resectoscopes in common use.

method of crushing bladder calculi. If the stones are larger than 2 cms the traditional blind lithotrite (Fig. 2.14), is inserted and the calculus crushed into pieces, which are small enough for the litholapaxy to be completed, under direct vision, with the cystoscopic lithotrite.

Cystoscopic foreign body removers

This is another instrument manufactured by Storz (Fig. 2.15), which has a limited, but definite use. It is introduced through a 26 charriére sheath and is used with a 70° telescope. Its function is to remove small foreign bodies or calculi. It can also be used for crushing

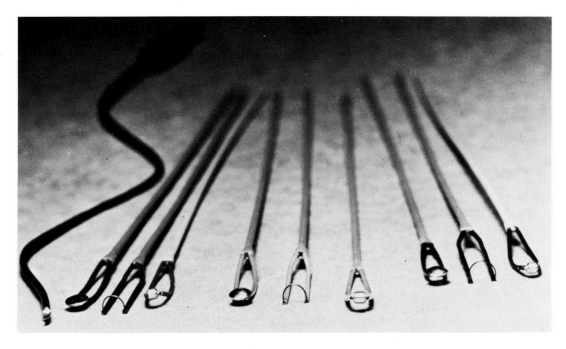

Fig. 2.12   Diathermy electrodes colour coded the same as the resectoscope sheaths.

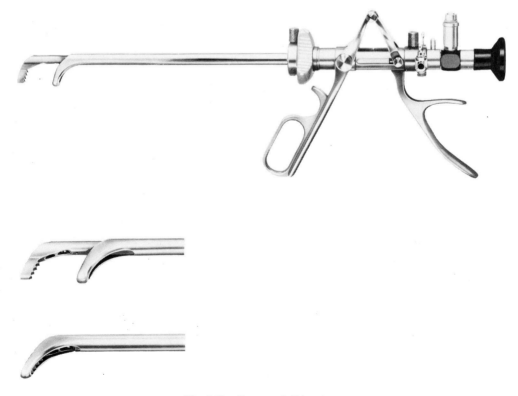

Fig. 2.13   Cystoscopic lithotrite.

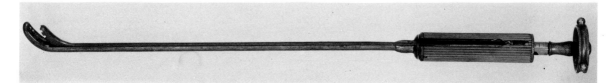

Fig. 2.14   Traditional blind lithotrite.

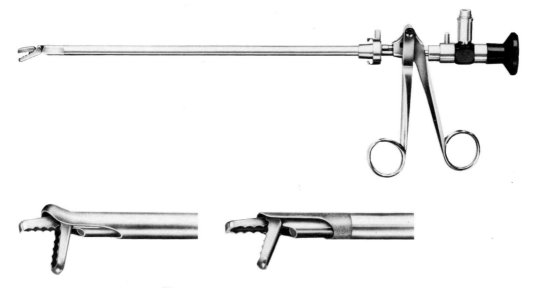

Fig. 2.15   Cystoscopic foreign body removers.

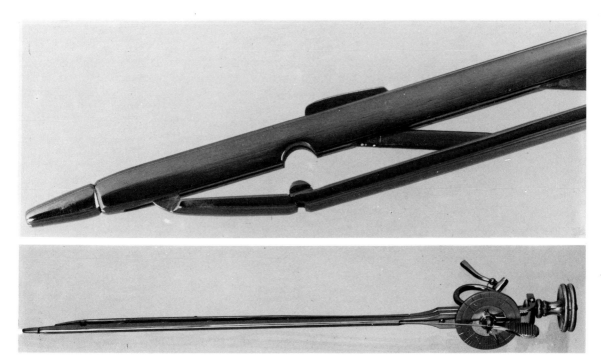

Figs. 2.16 and 2.17   Otis urethrotome (2 views).

small stones provided they are not too hard, as the construction is not so robust as the larger lithotrites.

Urethrotomy

The urethrotome is an indispensable item in the urologist's armamentarium. It can be used to calibrate the urethra, dilate the urethra prior to passing a cystoscope sheath, and to slit the urethra prior to carrying out an endoscopic resection. Emmert (1963) quoted the excellent results of preliminary internal urethrotomy, with an Otis urethrotome, in over a thousand cases of transurethral resection. It is not the usual practice in this country, but it is worth considering for use, in those patients whose urethra is narrow and has difficulty in accepting a 24 charriére sheath (Figs. 2.16 & 2.17).

Technique of endoscopic procedures

Position of the patient

One ideal position is for the patient to be placed flat on his back with his buttocks at the end of the table. Care should be taken to avoid a lithotomy position as this causes acute post-operative discomfort to the patient and is rarely any help to the operator. The hips should be flexed to an angle of about 45° and abducted to the same degree. Lloyd-Davies leg-supports are very satisfactory for achieving this position, as they readily adjust to the dimensions of each individual patient and ensure not only that there is pressure on the calves but also that the legs can be very readily readjusted in cases of osteoarthritis of the hip. Such a condition, can be quite impossible and the amount of abduction of the thigh obtained is insufficient to allow for adequate examination, let alone transurethral resection. In these cases transurethral resection has to be abandoned and replaced by an open surgical procedure (Fig. 2.18).

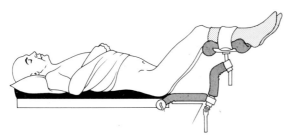

Fig. 2.18   Position of patient for endoscopic procedures.

Anaesthesia

The anaesthetic techniques used in endoscopic surgery are many and vary according to the procedure that is being adopted.

In the female, local anaesthetic is often satisfactory. If necessary, supplemented by 5–10 ml of intravenous

valium depending on the weight of the patient. Fifteen ml of 1 or 2 per cent lignocaine is instilled into the urethra using a urethral nozzle, the lignocaine being held in a vehicle, either a gel, glycerine or propylene glycol. It should remain about 5 minutes in the urethra before instrumentation commences. In the male, local anaesthesia is less popular owing to the length and confirmation of the urethra, but if used, about 20 ml of a similar solution is instilled and left for ten minutes prior to the start of the examination. Escape being avoided by either a penile clamp or digital compression.

It must not be forgotten that the comfort and peace of mind of the patient is all important and that a local anaesthetic should not be used in those patients who are apprehensive or who are worried about any discomfort or pain that may be associated with the examination. If the local is not used, the choice is between a general, and spinal or epidural. For a skilled anaesthetist there is very little difference between these two methods and it is better to have an experienced anaesthetist than to insist upon a special technique which is invariable. In no other surgery, is it more important to have a team of anaesthetist and surgeon, who are a regular partnership.

General anaesthesia can be extremely satisfactory especially if controlled hypotension is undertaken when necessary. In simple cystoscopic examinations, general anaesthesia may have to be used simply to alleviate the patient's anxiety and to ensure peace of mind. In these cases, scoline should be avoided, as patients may have quite severe muscle discomfort and pain for 24 hours afterwards.

The alternative to general anaesthesia is a spinal or epidural. An epidural is safer but it is time consuming, and is only satisfactory in about 85 per cent of cases and may be an extremely difficult procedure if a patient's spine is rigid and osteoarthritic. It has the advantage that the blood pressure can be controlled, because with an epidural, a catheter can be inserted into the epidural space and the anaesthetic topped up during the procedure, or even in the recovery ward so that the blood pressure is kept at a satisfactory level mark for a period of twelve hours and only slowly allowed to rise over this period. It cannot be too much emphasised, however, that if this technique is being used, the circulating blood volume must be kept normal, otherwise biochemical disturbances will take place. A spinal anaesthetic is very effective and does not cause undue delay, and produces adequate hypotension. However, disasters have occurred and because of this its popularity has waned and it is not often used. Nevertheless, the results are extremely good and it is a very satisfactory method for bladder tumour resections which are going to be prolonged and for prostate hypertrophy when up to 100 gms of tissue are being resected. In the excision of tumours and the prostate, hypotension is essential, if the best results are to be obtained. The choice of the method used must depend on the anaesthetist and the patient. Both drug induced hypertension and epidural or spinal anaesthesia can give very satisfactory control of blood pressure in the region of 80 or 90 mmHg. The tolerance that is accepted is diastolic minus 10 mmHg. It is not really necessary to go below this, as this level is very readily controlled and allows a rapid excision of large prostates.

Drug-induced hypotensive agents

The disadvantage here is that there is an extremely quick rise in the blood pressure at the end of the procedure. As a result it can cause rapid and excessive bleeding. Normally, this can be controlled by gentle contraction on the balloon of a foley catheter for 10 or 15 minutes.

Preparation of the urethra

It is good practice to use an antiseptic dissolved in a lubricant. There are many available but 0·5% chlorhexidine dissolved in either a gel, glycerine or propylene glycol is a satisfactory preparation. This can be either used from a tube or from a supply freshly prepared for each endoscopic session. For normal lubrication the above formulation is excellent but if local anaesthetic is required, in addition, then 1 or 2 per cent lignocaine can be added. The same solution can be used for lubricating instruments, but when employing resectoscopes it is a wise precaution to smear the shaft well with sterile vaseline.

Urethroscopy

A urethroscopy should never be considered an isolated examination but as part of a combined cystourethroscopy. In the female, a tight meatus may be present and require a simple dilatation with Hegars dilators, but rarely is a meatotomy required. The urethroscopy is carried out with either a 0° or 30° telescope. The sheath is initially inserted with the obturator *in situ* but once past the urethral orifice, the obturator is removed and is replaced by the telescope. Urethroscopy is always carried out with continuous irrigation. After inspection, palpation of the urethra through the vagina with the instrument *in situ* can be beneficial. In the male, a meatal stricture may also be present. It can be treated in one of three ways, simple dilatation, dorsal slit for 1 cm proximally from the meatus or dilatation with an Otis urethrotome with slits using the blade at 3 and 9 o'clock. This latter may be the most satisfactory method to prevent recurrent stricture. If it is the method employed, the urethral meatus should be dilated to 28 or 30 charriére before the slits are made. If the dorsal slit is used, it is important to stitch the urethral mucosa to the skin at the end of the endoscopic procedure. It is essential that the endoscope sheath passes the meatus without difficulty, as this is the most common place for recurrent strictures to be found.

Cystoscopy

The initial examination of the bladder should be carried out with the 30° telescope, the same instrument used for the urethroscopy. The same procedure is adopted in the male as in the female. The introducer being replaced by the telescope as soon as the tip enters the fossa navicularis. The instrument should never be forced, it should pass, largely by its own weight, and merely guided by the operator. The operator should familiarise himself with the normal bulbous, membranous and prostatic urethra including the verumontanum, the bladder neck and the external sphincter. For good vision, it is especially important in the male, to have satisfactory irrigating fluid which distends the urethra in front of the advancing telescope (Fig. 2.19).

It is fundamental that the operator adopts a technique which suits him and it must be one, which is repetitive, so that all areas of the bladder are seen. After the initial examination with a 30° telescope it should be replaced by the 70° so that areas on the roof particularly close to the bladder neck can be inspected. It is often helpful if light abdominal pressure is applied in the retropubic areas. This can be done, either by the operator or an assistant. This presses the bladder down into the view

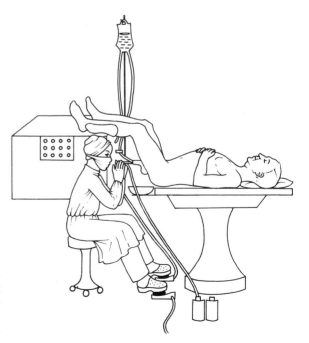

Fig. 2.19 Diagram of technique of using a continuous irrigating endoscope with fluid from the fluid producing machine.

of the telescope. Once the instrument has been passed into the bladder, the bladder should be emptied and the initial inspection carried out, as the bladder is filling. In this way small lesions can be observed, which otherwise might have been missed. There is no set technique in examining the bladder with a cystoscope. The examining surgeon must make his own plan and have a ritual, which he adheres to, for every examination. If there is any doubtful or suspicious lesion, particularly areas of inflammation in the bladder, a biopsy should be taken so that a precise diagnosis can be made. If a tumour is seen at the initial examination then the telescope and sheath are removed to be replaced by a resectoscope sheath and mechanisms are used to excise the tumour. The pieces are then sent for section for TNM grading.

Litholapaxy

The bladder is first washed out and filled with 200 ml of fluid. The instrument is lubricated and inserted with the jaws closed and locked. When the instrument enters the bladder the jaws are opened. When the blind instrument is being used, the handle is elevated and rotated through 90° and gently manipulated until the stone is engaged in the jaws. Before the stone is crushed the instrument is withdrawn slightly so that there is no contact with the bladder wall. This procedure is repeated until the fragments are small enough to be evacuated by either an Elick or Bigelow evacuator. The bladder must always be inspected with a cystoscopy at the end of the procedure to ensure that no fragments remain. If a cystoscopy lithotrite is being used, the calculus is engaged in the jaws and crushed under direct vision. As both these instruments are large (28 charriére) preliminary external meatotomy or urethral dilatation using the Otis urethrotome may be necessary.

Recently ultrasound has been used for litholapaxy. The basis of this method of treatment is that ultrasonic vibrations as a result of their high frequency 18–25000/sec are capable of giving up energy by direct contact with a solid object. In the case of ultrasonic litholapaxy, the vibration energy is directed into the bladder through a thin metal tube, the ultrasonic probe, which has an impact head. This probe is guided against the stone under direct vision through an endoscopic telescope (Fig. 2.20), as it is essential for the probe to be in direct contact with the stone. It is kept there by a vacuum produced in the probe tube, which sucks the stone against the tip. The ultrasonic vibrations are converted into powerful blows causing complete disintegration of the stone. This method is expensive and requires further evaluation before it can be recommended for general use. However, it is doubtful, in the present economic climate, whether it will ever be justified, except in special units which treat a large number of bladder stones.

Internal urethrotomy

Today internal urethrotomy has few indications and blind bouginage has been replaced by the threading of filiform bougies under direct vision through the stricture. In this way the stricture is dilated by screwing on to the filiform, bougies of gradually increasing calibre. Once the stricture has been dilated in this way an Otis urethrotomy can be passed and the stricture incised at 9 and 3 o'clock positions. To prevent rapid recurrence of such a stricture a silastic indwelling catheter should be passed and left for 2–3 weeks. In most cases this is only a palliative procedure, and the only real indication, is dilation of a narrow urethra in patients requiring a prostatic resection, litholapaxy or treatment for some other bladder pathology.

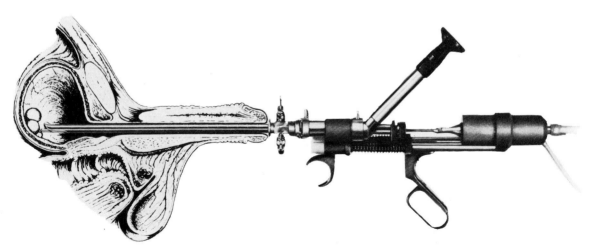

Fig. 2.20   Ultrasonic lithotrite manufactured by Storz.

Technique of resection of tumour

Small tumours present no problem. The bladder should be filled with 1·5 per cent glycine solution so that all rugi of the mucous membrane are flattened as, otherwise, there is always the risk of perforating the bladder. If the tumours are large, it is mandatory that the tumours should be resected from the periphery to the base and never initially cut off from the base, as if this happens, a large foreign body is left in the bladder which may not be able to pass through the urethra. This could lead to an embarrassing situation in which the bladder may well have to be opened. If the tumour is penetrating into, but not through the wall, the resection should be carried out, until normal muscle fibres are seen. If the tumour is penetrating through the muscle, then as much of the tumour as possible is resected. Clearly this type of tumour is beyond curative endoscopic surgery. An area of about 1 to 2 cms around a tumour should always be resected or coagulated by endoscopic diathermy, to destroy early malignant changes. Tumours on the roof may be difficult to excise and in these cases the best technique to adopt, is to carry out the resection while the bladder is slowly filling or when it is only partially filled. In some cases excision may still be impossible and abdominal pressure forcing the fundus of the bladder down towards the operator is invaluable. When the tumours are on the fundus of the bladder, close to the bladder neck, it may be necessary to excise part of the bladder neck or in the male, a considerable part of the roof of the prostate, to achieve satisfactory access.

Endoscopic resection of the prostate

It is not the purpose of this book to describe the expertise required for endoscopic resection of the prostate, as it has been well-documented in many other books. Suffice to say that, it is most important to carry out a preliminary urethroscopy so that a coincidental urethral lesion can be excluded. In addition to the urethroscopy the bladder should be thoroughly inspected to exclude coexisting bladder pathology.

Both of these examinations are important as the best method of treatment will be decided on the findings. If a bladder tumour, diverticula or large calculus is discovered open operation should be performed, but if there is no serious bladder pathology then transurethral resection of the prostate is the best method, provided the gland is not too large.

Rectal examination should never be omitted. It is performed with and without the endoscope in the urethra, the latter being most important as it will give valuable information on the size of the apical and lateral lobes.

As a satisfactory system for the continuous production of sterile, pyrogen-free, low mineral content water, there has now been produced (Chapter 7) an irrigating endoscopic system, which is the logical development to utilise its full potential. Such a system embracing simultaneous irrigation, suction and low intravesical pressure has been produced by Iglesias. This will allow an uninterrupted resection, apart from the evacuation of the resected pieces of tissue, less operating time, and the reduction in the amount of fluid absorbed during the resection. This method must ultimately, become the standard technique.

REFERENCES

Emmett, J. L., Rouse, S. N., Green, L. F., De Weerd, J. H. and Utz, D. C. (1963). Preliminary internal urethrotomy in 1036 cases, to prevent urethral stricture following transurethral resection. Calibre of normal adult male urethra. *Journal of Urology*, **89**, 329.

Iglesias, J. J. (1973). Iglesias resectoscope with simultaneous irrigation, suction and low intravesical pressure. Department of Surgery, Division of Urology, College of Medicine and Dentistry of New Jersey and Affiliated Hospitals, New Jersey Medical School.

3. The modern urological endoscope

Professor H. H. Hopkins, F.R.S.

Introduction

The optical performance of medical endoscopes has been improved many-fold during the last two decades. The invention of fibre-optics (Hopkins and Kapany, 1954; Van Heel, 1954) has led to highly flexible endoscopes which permit routine examination and clinical procedures in practically the whole of the digestive tract. In urology, and other disciplines which use rigid endoscopes, fibre-optics has replaced the former distal lamp and has made possible the use of external light sources of high intensity and colour temperature. The arrangement is shown diagrammatically in Figures 3.1 and 3.2. With a modern cystoscope the illumination of the bladder wall can thereby be intense enough, and sufficiently 'white', for both still and ciné colour photography.

The second step in development, was the invention of the Hopkins rod-lens system for rigid endoscopes (Hopkins, 1960). The traditional telescope, shown schematically in Figure 3.3, employed a group of lenses, constituting an objective, followed by a succession of relay systems. The rôle of the objective is to produce at 0_1 a reduced image of the observed object at 0. The first relay system re-images 0_1 at 0_2, and in the same manner the succeeding relay systems carry the image to the proximal end of the endoscope, where it is magnified by the eyepiece before reaching the eye of the observer.

So-called field lenses have to be placed at each intermediate image, as at 0_1 and 0_2 in the upper diagram. If these lenses were not there, the pencils of light coming from the preceeding objectives to form the images of extra-axial points of the object would continue to diverge and be reflected at the inner wall of the containing tube. Each field lens system forms an image of the preceeding relay objective at the following relay system, thereby ensuring that all rays leaving the former are refracted to pass through the latter.

In the new system the image is relayed by a succession of rod-lenses, as illustrated in Figure 3.3. The traditional system consisted of a tube of air with thin lenses of glass. By contrast, the new system may be regarded as a tube of glass with thin lenses of air. The rôles of the objective and eyepiece in rod-lens systems are essentially the same as in the traditional system. In practice, there will be typically five relay stages in a cystoscope, rather than only two as in the schematic diagrams of Figure 3.3.

The effect of using glass-spaces and air-lenses, in place of air-space and glass-lenses, is twofold. Optically the total light transmitted is increased by a factor n^2, where n is the refractive index of the glass used for the rod lenses. The value of n^2 can lie between $(1 \cdot 50)^2 = 2 \cdot 25$ and $(1 \cdot 65)^2 = 2 \cdot 72$. Mechanically, the ease and precision of mounting of the rod lenses permits a greater diameter to be used for the lenses for a given outer diameter of the telescope. In the first prototype to be constructed this radius of clear aperture was increased by a factor $1 \cdot 4$, giving an increase in transmission by a factor $(1 \cdot 4)^4 = 3 \cdot 8$. Taken together these two factors gave an increased transmission of about nine times. Subsequent, commercially produced, cystoscopes employed this advantage to give both smaller outside diameter and a field of view of 70° compared with the more typical value of 40° for traditional cystoscopes.

A third factor, which contributes notably to the brightness and contrast of the image in the modern endoscope, is the use of efficient multi-layer anti-reflection coatings on the surfaces of the lenses. When light enters or leaves a lens with untreated surfaces, between four and six per cent of the light is reflected backwards. With, typically, more than 40 air/glass surfaces in a telescope, this results in a serious loss of light. Some of this reflected light is also reflected forwards again by each of the preceeding surfaces, giving either a general haze or glare over the image, which significantly reduces the contrast between the darker and brighter parts, or ghost images may be formed. Simple blooming of the type now commonly used for ordinary camera lenses reduces this effect: multilayer coatings give a further improvement. Typical transmission figures for a system having 40 air/glass surfaces would be:

untreated surfaces   10 per cent,
bloomed surfaces   70 per cent,
multilayer coatings   90 per cent.

This alone can give a nine times improvement in transmission over earlier endoscopes, which had to use untreated lenses. Taken together, with the transmission advantages of the rod-lens systems, the modern rod-lens cystoscope can have a total light transmission some 80

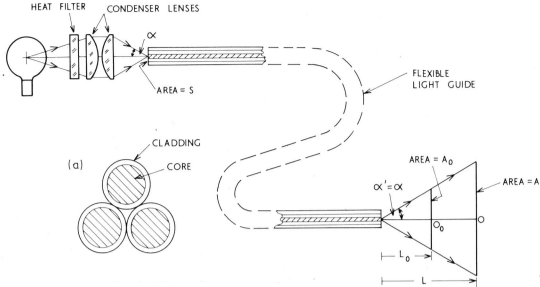

Fig. 3.1   Light source and fibre optic light guide.

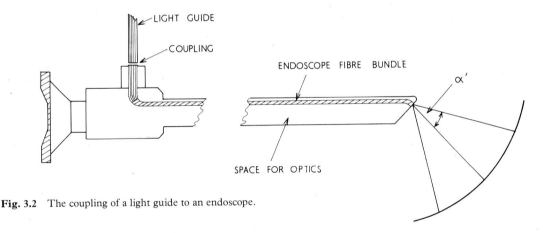

Fig. 3.2   The coupling of a light guide to an endoscope.

times greater than a pre-war traditional system of the same external diameter.

Finally, it should be said, that modern research on the theory of the formation of optical images revealed, surprisingly, that the design of the optical system and the precision of manufacture both required the same high standards as those demanded by a good quality microscope objective. The use of computers has contributed significantly to the optical design, and much more precise assembly is possible using rod lenses.

Illuminating systems

The components of the illuminating system of a modern endoscope are:

1. a light source,
2. a condenser system with heat filter,
3. a flexible light guide (i.e. a light cable),

C

4. a fibre bundle in the endoscope itself.

These are shown in Figures 3.1 and 3.2 respectively.

The light source

For routine examination a quartz-iodine lamp is usually employed. This is a tungsten filament lamp, which can be run at higher brightness and colour temperature than a normal tungsten lamp. For still photography, a flash tube, usually of about 300 joules, is employed. This may either be placed in the light source housing, with the light fed to the endoscope by means of the usual light cable, or a special flash unit, of the kind described later, fixes directly on the endoscope and feeds straight into the endoscope's fibre bundle shown in Figure 3.2.

For ciné-photography, or when the image is to be conveyed to a television camera for display on a remote monitor, a high power xenon arc is used. Typically,

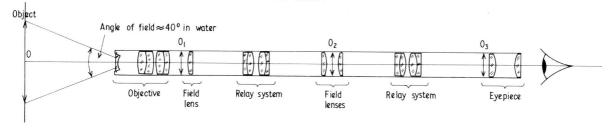

(a) TRADITIONAL SYSTEM

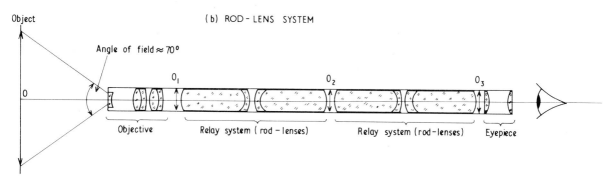

(b) ROD - LENS SYSTEM

Fig. 3.3   Schematic diagrams of the optics of a traditional cystoscope and of a rod-lens system.

the power consumption of this will be 2000 watts, and it gives a very high intrinsic luminosity together with a high colour temperature.

It may seem surprising that such high powers are needed in the light sources employed in cystoscopy, where an area of, say, only 30 mm diameter is to be illuminated. The reasons lie in the light losses in the different parts of the illuminating system, in the small diameter imposed on the endoscope fibre bundle, and in the small aperture that may be allowed to the endoscope itself consistent with there being an adequate depth of focus. The light source must also have a high colour temperature, so that the light is not deficient in blue. This is because good colour rendering is needed in the images of objects in which the detail, so often, consists of small differences in colour rather than differences in brightness, and also because light in the blue end of the visible spectrum is absorbed more in traversing the glass of the light guides than that in the green and red parts of the spectrum.

The condenser system

The condenser lenses, shown merely schematically in Figure 3.1, form an image of the light source on the proximal end of the light cable. They have to be high aperture lenses similar to the condenser system used in a slide projector. The aperture angle α, shown in Figure 3.1, may be larger than 30°. One or more heat filters are provided, but, even so, the heat reaching the end of the

light cable may sometimes be sufficient to cause damage.

An alternative arrangement, shown in Figure 3.4, employs a concave mirror for imaging the light source on the light cable. A so-called cold mirror is employed, the reflecting surface consisting of a thin-film multi-layer, which can have a reflectance of only 20 per cent for infra-red radiation and a reflectance of 95 per cent for the visible part of the spectrum. Most of the heat-radiation is thus not reflected.

The light cable

The fibre-optic light cable consists of a large number of glass fibres, as suggested in Figure 3.1. Each fibre in the

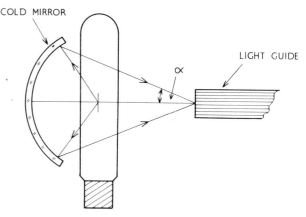

Fig. 3.4   The use of a dichroic (cold) mirror.

bundle consists of a core of glass of high refractive index with a thin cladding of glass of lower refractive index, as shown in Figure 3.1. Light falling on the core of any fibre suffers repeated reflections at the fibre wall; the entering light is thereby trapped and is transmitted to the distal end of the given fibre. Light falling on the claddings, or on the interstices between the fibres, is not trapped: it is eventually lost by absorption at the plastic sheath surrounding the bundle. The active area of the bundle of fibres is, thus, only that of the fibre cores, which occupies about 70 per cent of the total area of the bundle. The effective transmittance of the entry face of the bundle takes account of this so-called packing-fraction, and of the loss of reflection at the air-glass interface which may amount to 6 per cent. The effective transmittance of this interface is, therefore, only about 66 per cent.

The overall transmittance of the light cable is further reduced by absorption as the light travels through the fibre, and also by a second 6 per cent reflection loss at the distal exit-face of the fibre bundle. For a good quality fibre bundle, the result is to give an overall transmit-

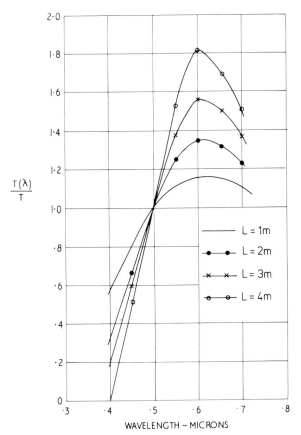

Fig. 3.5 The ratio of the overall transmittance of a fibre bundle for different wavelengths to the overall transmittance for white light.

tance for white light of about 50 per cent for a light cable of 1 metre length. For longer light cables, it is only the absorption in the greater length of glass which gives an increased loss of light, and it is found that a 2 metre light cable can have a white light transmittance of about 40 per cent.

Of the above sources of light loss, only the absorption in the glass depends on the wavelength of the light, it being appreciably greater for the blue end of the visible spectrum. The result is that with increasing length of the fibre bundle there is not only some decrease in overall transmittance, but, more seriously, an increasing relative depletion of blue in the light emerging. Unless a source of high colour temperature is used, the light leaving the light cable has a yellowish appearance, which is greater, the longer the cable. Figure 3.5 illustrates the effect; the visible region of the spectrum extending from the extreme blue at 0.4μ to the red at 0.7μ.

Since the object of the light cable is merely to convey light from the proximal to the distal end there is no need for the fibres in the bundle to be in corresponding order at the two ends of the bundle. This is termed an incoherent bundle. In a flexible fibre-optic endoscope the bundle of fibres has to be ordered in such a manner that the position of each fibre at the distal end corresponds with its position at the proximal end of the bundle. This, known as a coherent bundle, is the type of fibre-optic unit employed in the modern gastroscope and in fibre-optic teaching attachments. The need for exact ordering is why an image bundle, that is a coherent bundle, is so much more expensive than the incoherent bundles used as light cables. Furthermore, the useful life of a coherent bundle is much less than that of an incoherent bundle, because in the latter case the presence of broken fibres will merely reduce the light transmission, whereas with a coherent bundle the breakage of an appreciable number of fibres produces a corresponding set of black dots which seriously impairs the appearance of the image.

The endoscope fibre bundle
As shown in Figure 3.2, the light cable is made to abut on a fibre bundle incorporated in the endoscope itself. There are light losses at this coupling arising from three separate causes. Two of these are illustrated in Figure 3.6, where bundle 1 is the light cable, and bundle 2 is the light guide in the endoscope. In Figure 3.6, there is a finite separation between the abutting ends of the two bundles; and, as shown by the hatched regions, some of the light emerging from the fibres of bundle 1 falls outside the entry face of bundle 2. These losses may, of course, be reduced to a negligible amount merely by ensuring close contact between the two bundles. The second cause of light loss is the 6 per cent reflection of light at each of the two abutting air/glass

(a)

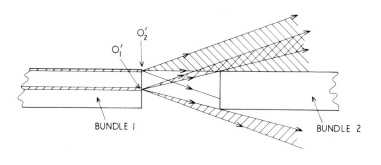

(b)

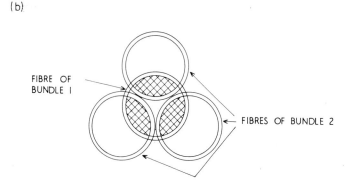

Fig. 3.6   Light losses on coupling two light guides. (a) Separation effect. (b) Mismatch.

interfaces. Finally there is mismatch between the individual fibres of the two bundles, as illustrated in Figure 3.6. This is the worst case, where a fibre of bundle 1 has its centre opposite the interstice of three fibres of bundle 2. Of the light emerging from the bundle 1 fibre, only that which is incident on the cores of the bundle 2 fibres is transmitted. For randomly arranged fibres, the degree of overlap of corresponding fibre ends will range from that shown in Figure 3.6 to perfect coincidence. The overall degree of overlap is estimated at about 80 per cent. If the two reflection losses are included, the overall transmittance of such a coupling between two light guides is about 70 per cent.

We now come to a factor which is peculiar to cystoscopy, or to any wide-angle endoscope working in water. In Figure 3.1, a cone of light of semi-angle α falls on the proximal end of the light cable. As shown in the particular diagram it is assumed that the light emerges into air, where it leaves the fibre as a cone, which is also of semi-angle $\alpha' = \alpha$. The light rays are less inclined to the axis when in the fibre, because of refraction at the entry face; this inclination is then returned to its entering value by refraction out of the fibre into air. When the light emerges into water there is much less refraction of the rays, so that the angle α' of the emergent cone is less than the angle α of the incident cone.

The situation is illustrated in Figure 3.7, where cones of semi-angles $\alpha = 38°$ and $\alpha = 53°$ are shown entering

1. a low aperture fibre
2. a high aperture fibre respectively.

When emerging into air, these give $\alpha' = 38°$ and $\alpha' = 53°$ but only values $\alpha' = 27°$ and $\alpha' = 37°$ when the light emerges into water. For this reason, high-aperture fibres must be used in the endoscope bundle when the field of 70° of a modern cystoscope has to be illuminated. Now present-day high aperture fibres have greater absorption in the blue end of the visible spectrum, and to reduce such losses the light cable is usually made using low-aperture fibres. It is then necessary to increase the cone angle of the illumination. This is achieved by the use of a fibre cone, between the light cable 1 and the endoscope bundle 2, as illustrated in Figure 3.8, the increase in the aperture being inversely proportional to the reduction in diameter.

If the fibre cone is cemented to the proximal entry face of the endoscope bundle, shown as bundle 2 in

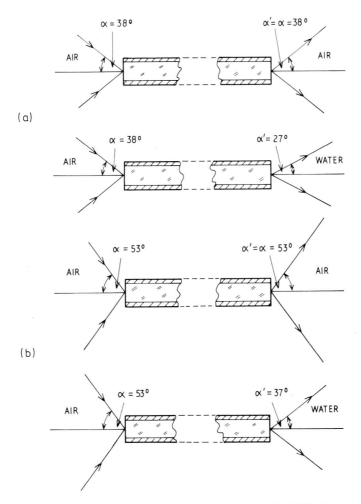

(a)

(b)

Fig. 3.7 Fibres feeding into air and water. (a) Low aperture fibre: $n = 1.64$, $n' = 1.52$. (b) High aperture fibre: $n = 1.72$, $n' = 1.52$.

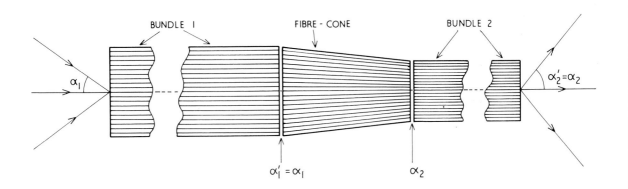

Fig. 3.8 The use of a conical fibre bundle to couple two light guides (schematic).

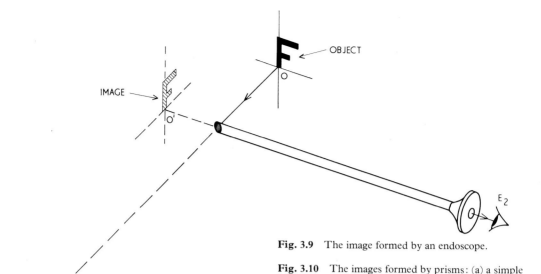

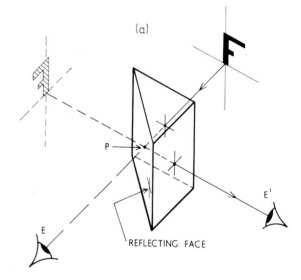

Fig. 3.9 The image formed by an endoscope.

Fig. 3.10 The images formed by prisms: (a) a simple reflecting prism; (b) an Amici roof prism.

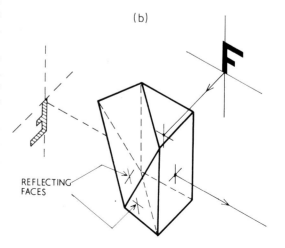

Figure 3.8, there will be a transmittance of about 80% across the interface, the loss being then due only to mismatch of the fibres.

Assuming a 2-metre long light cable (transmittance = 40 per cent), which couples (with a transmittance = 70 per cent) to a fibre cone cemented to the endoscope bundle (coupling transmittance = 80 per cent), there will be only 22 per cent of the light falling on the proximal end of the cable which is transmitted to illuminate the object. In practical systems, the amount of light transmitted may be even less than this estimated value of 22 per cent.

Endoscopes employing rod-lenses

The function of the endoscope itself is to render the interior of the body cavity observable to the endoscopist exactly as if it were being viewed by him directly. This is illustrated in Figure 3.9, where the object is the letter F at the 0: the image has to be formed at $0'$ when the object is viewed by an observer at E_2 using a right-angle endoscope. This observer requires to see exactly what an observer at E_1 would see when viewing the object directly. This requires that the image of the letter F be seen correctly top-to-bottom and also left-to-right. For any, other than a forward-viewing, endoscope reflecting prisms are used to deviate the optical axis, as shown in Figures 3.10 and 3.11. To avoid a mirror image, whose form is ꟻ not F, there must be an even number of reflections in the optical system overall.

Figure 3.10 shows a simple right-angle reflecting prism which, placed at the distal end of the endoscope, gives a mirror-type image as shown in Figure 3.10. Such

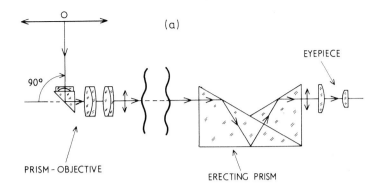

(a)

EYEPIECE

90°

PRISM - OBJECTIVE

ERECTING PRISM

(b)

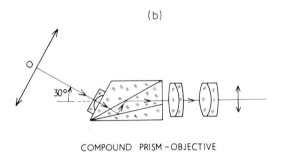

30°

COMPOUND PRISM - OBJECTIVE

Fig. 3.11 Prism-objectives giving different viewing directions: (a) $= 90°$; (b) $= 30°$.

a view would be hopelessly confusing; and, to correct it, earlier instruments used the Amici prism shown in Figure 3.10. The image seen is now ꓸ; and, if a lens system forms an inverted image of this, the final view seen is correctly F.

The so-called roof edge on an Amici prism has serious practical difficulties in the small sizes needed for endoscopes. In the right-angle viewing cystoscope designed by Hopkins the better arrangement shown in Figure 3.11 was adopted, with a simple reflecting prism incorporated as part of the objective. The image is then corrected at the proximal end of the endoscope by means of an erecting prism, as shown. For the 30° fore-oblique instrument, two reflections are used, as shown in Figure 3.11. In this case, the final image is formed correctly, without any resultant mirror-inversion. The compound prism used here is again built into the objective assembly.

In both cases, the objective forms a reduced image, as at 0_1 for the direct viewing system shown in Figure 3.3. The relay systems, usually five in number, then successively re-image 0_1 to give a final image, as at 0_3 in Figure 3.3. This is then magnified by the eyepiece to give the final view to the endoscopist. The advantages

of adopting the rod-lens principle have already been mentioned in the introduction above. The increase in the total light transmitted was there attributed to two causes. The first is fundamental, deriving from the basic laws of image formation in optics, from which it may be shown that the total light transmission is increased by a factor equal to the square of the refractive index of the glass used for the rod-lenses.

The second factor derives from the simpler mechanical construction made possible by the use of rod-lenses in place of the ordinary lenses of the traditional system. The methods of mounting the lenses in the endoscope tube are illustrated in Figure 3.12. For a given outside diameter, the radius of clear aperture ρ_2 with rod lenses is greater than the radius ρ_1 for the traditional system. This gives an increase in the total light transmitted by a factor of $(\rho_2/\rho_1)^4$, so that a 20% increase in radius of clear aperture gives the large increase of 107% in the light which can be transmitted.

It may be noted that it was the increased light transmitting power, and the possibility of simple and very precise assembly, offered by the rod-lens principle, that made possible the realisation of the first satisfactory infant cystoscopes.

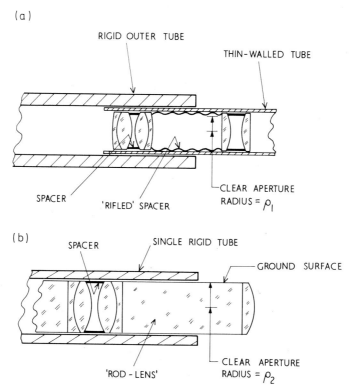

Fig. 3.12   The mechanical construction of: (a) the traditional endoscope, and (b) the new system.

The light accepted by the endoscope from the illuminated object is illustrated in Figure 3.13. Rays from each fibre of the bundle fall on any point such as 0, where the light is reflected. There is usually diffuse reflection, and usually only a relatively small part of the reflected light is accepted by the observing endoscope, as shown by the accepted cone in the diagram. Even under favourable circumstances, the total light accepted from all points of the object may be less than 10% of that emerging from the fibre bundle. Moreover, this fraction of the light which is accepted by the endoscope decreases inversely as the square of the distance of the object from the distal end of the fibre bundle.

In Figure 3.1, for example, the areas of the circular patches illuminated at the distances L and L_0 from the distal end of the endoscope bundle are in the ratio $A/A_0 = (L/L_0)^2$. Since a given total amount of light is spread over the larger area A, the intensities of illumination of the two planes will be in the inverse ratio $(L_0/L)^2$. This relation assumes that the diameter of the fibre bundle is small, compared with the distances L and L_0, but in practical cases the error is rarely more than a few per cent.

This decrease in illumination is very obvious in observation use when the endoscope is withdrawn to a greater distance. It is a serious factor in photography, where if the distance from the object is doubled the exposure needs to be increased fourfold to compensate for the decrease in light accepted by the endoscope.

The magnification of an endoscope also decreases in inverse proportion to the distance of the object. The object field angle is constant, and this is reproduced as a fixed apparent angular size when observed through the eyepiece. Thus, for an object at greater distance, a

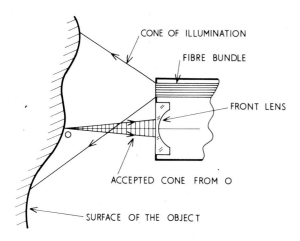

Fig. 3.13   The light accepted by an endoscope.

larger diameter of the object is seen, by the observer to be of the same angular size. That is, the magnification is reduced, and the smallest detail in the object that can be resolved, is also correspondingly larger.

In the interests of sterilisation it is desirable to avoid moving parts on the cystoscope itself. It is for this reason that no provision is made for focusing, and depth of focus has to be relied upon to see objects at different distances. For a typical specification of operating cystoscope, if the instrument is in exact focus for a given observer when the object is at a distance L = 20 mm, there will, theoretically, be almost perfect definition in the range from L = 7 mm to L = 33 mm. For younger observers, this range of good focus can be extended by the exercise of visual accommodation, but this becomes increasingly reduced with age. The result is that adequately good definition is usually possible over the whole range of distances which occur in practice. It is nevertheless desirable to have a focusing facility on photographic and television cameras when used with endoscopes, and also for dual-viewing (i.e. teaching) attachments.

Again, for a typical operating cystoscope, the smallest resolved detail in the object, when exactly focused with the object at L = 20 mm, under ideal conditions, is approximately 0·05 mm. This can be rarely achieved in practice, and a safer rule-of-thumb limit is 0·10 mm. For a 70° angle of field, having a diameter of 28 mm for L = 20 mm, this gives the smallest resolved detail as about $\frac{1}{300}$th of the image diameter. This figure may also be used for, either the visual image, or for a photograph, although definition is inevitably lost in photography. Moreover, even visually, the expected resolution is smaller towards the edge of the image. In all cases, however, the definition obtainable is greatly superior to the best which is possible with fibre-optic endoscopes.

Dual-viewing (teaching) attachments

A dual-viewing attachment is a device which may be attached to the eyepiece of an endoscope in order to provide a viewing point for a second observer. This observer then sees exactly what the endoscopist is observing. The uses of such an attachment are three-fold. First they may be used for teaching, either with the student observing a procedure carried out by the instructor, or *vice-versa*, with the instructor monitoring or directing the carrying out of a procedure by the student. Second, a dual-viewing attachment used for observation may be employed, when the endoscopist wishes to consult a colleague. Third, a camera may be used at the proximal end of the attachment in order to carry out photography for documentation, or for a television transmission, without interfering with the routine of the endoscopist.

Because of the need for flexibility, the first dual-viewing devices were fibre-optic systems. The basic principle is illustrated in Figure 3.14. The beam-splitting cube has a partially-reflecting/partially-transmitting diagonal face. For visual observation the beam-splitter has approximately equal transmittance and reflectance: for still or ciné photography, or for television, a reflectance of about 90 per cent with a low transmittance is preferable. An objective at the distal end of the attachment receives the light reflected from the beam-splitter, and forms an image at the plane 0. This image is conveyed to the plane 0′, by means of a fibre-bundle (or by a lens and prism system, as described below), where an eyepiece at the proximal end magnifies the image at 0′ for viewing by the second observer.

A typical length for fibre-optic teaching attachments is 500 mm, with an external diameter of about 10 mm and a high degree of flexibility along the whole length. They are light in weight, and scarcely impede at all, the procedure of an endoscopy. Their disadvantages are poor image quality, and the deterioration of the image-transporting bundle because of damaged or broken fibres which result from repeated flexures of the device. Replacement fibre-bundles are very costly.

The relatively poor image quality of the fibre-optic teaching attachment arises principally from two causes. To transport an image, as from 0 to 0′ in Figure 3.14, a coherent fibre-bundle has to be used. In this the fibres require to have the same ordering at the two ends of the bundle. Light falling on the fibre at 0 is trapped in this fibre and appears as a dot of light at 0′, the proximal end of the fibre. The image thus consists of an array of dots, each of an intensity and colour corresponding to the light falling on the distal end of the given fibre. The smallest diameter of fibre used is about 10μ: for a fibre of smaller diameter, so-called wave-guide effects occur and light leaks out of the fibre. A useful practical rule gives the value 2·5d for the resolution limit of a coherent fibre-bundle, where d = fibre diameter. This is a factor of 2 to 3 times coarser than the resolution limit of a corresponding lens system. Thus, even with perfect focusing of the image at 0, and with a perfect bundle, there is an appreciable loss of resolution in the image seen by the second observer.

In addition to the above effect, arising from the discrete structure of the fibre-optic image, any error of focus of the image 0 at the proximal end of the fibre bundle means that light from a single point of the endoscope image, which should fall on only one fibre, falls on several adjacent fibres. No re-focusing at the proximal end can correct this, and the image is irretrievably blurred. The eyepiece of the attachment may be made focusable, but this serves merely to bring the proximal end of the fibre-bundle into good focus: it cannot take light emerging from several adjacent fibres and make it appear to come from a single fibre.

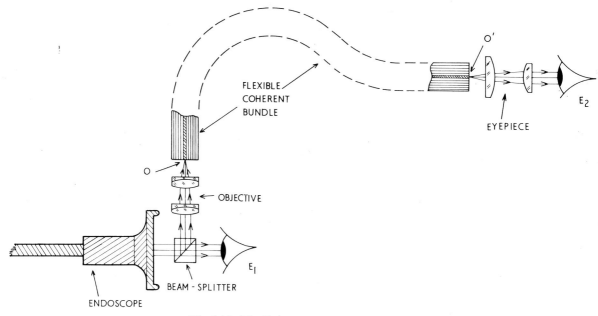

Fig. 3.14   The fibre-optic teaching attachment.

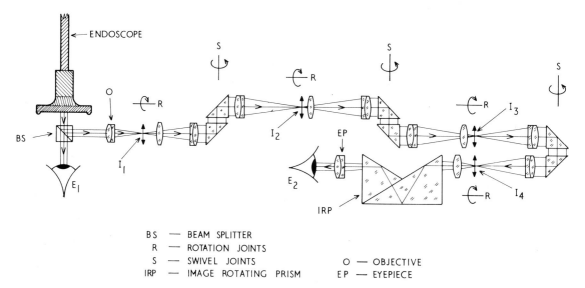

BS	—	BEAM SPLITTER
R	—	ROTATION JOINTS
S	—	SWIVEL JOINTS
IRP	—	IMAGE ROTATING PRISM

O — OBJECTIVE
EP — EYEPIECE

Fig. 3.15   A dual-viewing attachment (Schematic).

By contrast, the image seen in the lens-type attachment, to be described later, may be very accurately focused by means of the proximal eyepiece.

The above two effects are alone sufficient to explain the poorer image quality obtained with a fibre-optic dual-viewing attachment. To these must be added, the presence of misalignment of fibres, which occurs in all but the very best bundles, and the presence of broken fibres which studs the image with small black dots.

Figure 3.15 illustrates the construction adopted for a lens and prism type of dual-viewing attachment.* It employs a beam-splitter and objective 0, which forms an image at 0_1. This image is then relayed, by means of a train of lenses and prisms, to the proximal end where it is magnified by an eyepiece EP for viewing by the second observer at E_2. The overall length of the

*This system was designed, and prototypes produced by a small Medical Optics Unit in the Physics Department, University of Reading, financed by the Department of Health and Social Security.

attachment is 930 mm, and each of the several sections is contained in light alloy tubes of 20 mm diameter. It is an articulated system, with swivel joints permitting full 360° rotations at the points marked S in Figure 3.15, and each tube is in two halves with rotation joints at the points marked R. The result is a high degree of flexibility, but not, of course, as full as the continuous flexibility offered by a fibre-optic system.

Incorporated in the eyepiece EP is a prism IRP, the rotation of which, rotates the image seen by the second observer, permitting him to orient it as desired. The eyepiece is focusable; and, since no reliance need now be placed on depth of focus for observing objects at different distances, very sharp focus may be achieved for any object. In practical use the second observer frequently sees, in consequence, a sharper image than the endoscopist. With regard to weight and continuous flexibility the advantage lies with fibre-optic teaching attachments. However, the much superior image quality and there being no need for replacement of expensive fibre-bundles gives an overwhelming advantage to the lens and mirror-articulated type of attachment. Simple dual-viewing attachments consisting of a single rigid arm incorporating lens systems have also been made.

Endoscopic photography

To photograph or film an endoscope image the camera may be attached either directly to the endoscope, or to the proximal eyepiece of a dual-viewing attachment. The latter method has the advantage that the camera may be left permanently in position, and need not interrupt the endoscopic examination. If the camera is used directly on the endoscope there is not only an interruption for the endoscopist, but the area to be photographed has to be found again.

An ordinary 35 mm camera may be used, as shown schematically in Figure 3.16. A typical focal length required for the lens is 75 mm, giving an image of about 12 mm in diameter, but a zoom objective having a focal length range from about 120 mm to 40 mm, giving image diameters in the range 7 mm to 22 mm, is an advantage. The reason for this is as follows. The total amount of light leaving the endoscope is clearly not affected by the focal length of the camera lens. Now the diameter of the image produced on the film is directly proportional to the focal length of the lens employed; so that, the area of the image being proportional to the square of its diameter, the intensity of illumination falling on the film is inversely proportional to the square of the focal length. Thus, a shorter focal length produces a smaller size of image but a brighter one. In consequence, if the focal length is changed from 120 mm to 40 mm, the necessary exposure time is reduced by the factor $(40/120)^2 = 1/9$. This possibility is frequently of great advantage in endoscopic photography, where there is so often a shortage of light in the image.

If a shorter focal length camera lens, or the short focal length of a zoom objective, is employed, the same diameter of the object is merely reproduced on a smaller scale, on the film. There is an increase in brightness of the image, but the detail appears on a smaller scale. No resolution is lost provided the film will resolve it. Increased brightness of the image may also be obtained by decreasing the distance of the distal end of the endoscope from the object being observed. In this case a smaller region of the object is seen; it is reproduced with the same size on the film, and the detail is correspondingly larger. It is often necessary in endoscopic photography to use one, or both, of the above methods for increasing the brightness of the

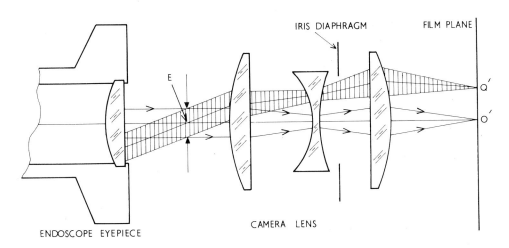

Fig. 3.16 Ray paths in endoscopic photography.

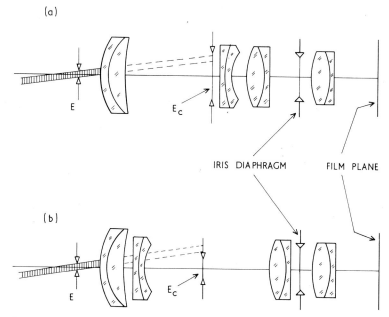

Fig. 3.17 A zoom camera objective, showing vignetting of an endoscopic image. (a) = long-focus position. (b) = short-focus position.

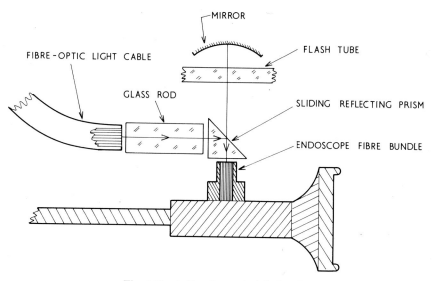

Fig. 3.18 A directly attached flash unit.

image in order to overcome a shortage of light.

The pencils of light from the different points of a cystoscope image emerge, as shown in Figure 3.16 through an exit pupil E, whose diameter is typically around 2 mm. A lens of focal length 75 mm, thus works at an F/ratio of F/32·5, which is extremely small. It is, nevertheless, usually necessary to work with the iris diaphragm fully open. This is because pencils of light, such as that forming the off-axis image point Q′ in the diagram, and shown shaded, pass eccentrically through

the iris diaphragm of the camera lens. Reducing the size of opening can cut off some of the light beams forming the outer parts of the image. This vignetting of the image may happen if an ordinary zoom objective is used, even with the iris diaphragm fully open. This is because, as illustrated in Figure 3.17, the iris diaphragm is then even further from the front of the objective. For both fixed and zoom objectives, vignetting is more likely to occur if the front surface is placed too far from the endoscope eyepiece.

Much simpler camera lenses, both fixed focus and zoom lenses, have been especially designed for endoscopic photography. These are, in many ways, much to be preferred over ordinary camera lenses.

Focussing of the image is essential for good endoscopic photography. If the camera is used directly on the cystoscope, this has to be achieved by focussing the camera lens. When photography is carried out using a dual-viewing attachment, the camera lens may be set for infinity and focussing is then achieved by means of the proximal eyepiece of the attachment.

For ciné photography, and for television, a continuously running high power light source, usually a xenon arc, is necessary. For still photography, various electronic flash units are available. The requirement here is for there to be adequate illumination for observation through the camera view-finder, and to feed all of the light from the flash to the endoscope bundle during the exposure.

A flash source may be built into a console housing several other sources, each of which may be fed at choice by way of the ordinary light cable to the endoscope. Alternatively a flash unit may be attached to the endoscope, as shown diagrammatically in Figure 3.18. This particular unit* has a reflecting prism, which in the position shown reflects light from the ordinary light cable, by way of a glass rod, to the endoscope fibre bundle. In this position there is the ordinary illumination for visual observation. To take a photograph a flash release cable is pressed, which first moves the prism downwards to allow the flash tube to be imaged directly on to the endoscope bundle by means of the concave mirror shown. At the end of its traverse, the prism slide actuates the flash for taking the photograph.

In black and white photography there is considerable latitude allowed for the exposure. For satisfactory colour photography much less latitude may be allowed, and some photometric control over the exposure is desirable. Cameras, and flash units, are fortunately now available with exposure control as a built-in facility.

*Designed in the Medical Optics Units at Reading University: patents applied for.

REFERENCES

Hopkins, H. H. and Kapany, N. S. *Nature*, Vol. **173**, p. 39 Jan. 2, 1954.
van Heel, A. C. S. *Nature*, Vol. **173**, p. 39, Jan. 2, 1954.
British Patent No. 954629, 1960.

4. Photography

Endoscopic photography should now be accepted as part of urological technology and photographic equipment ought always to be available to record pathological changes in the bladder. These photographs can be kept as a record in the case sheet and can be used at any time to compare bladder lesions with those taken on all previous occasions. One of the authors (J. G. Gow), became interested in the subject over twenty years ago, when he attempted to take photographs through the cystoscopic telescopes in use at that time. The results were unsuccessful, owing to the poor optical systems and the inadequacy of the light intensity in the bladder. About this time, Hopkins working at Imperial College, was approached and he agreed to institute a programme of investigation aimed at improving the optical system of the telescope. These investigations showed that the optical system in the telescope was quite inadequate for many reasons, and however well made, would not be good enough to allow satisfactory pictures to be taken. Hopkins then designed the Hopkins Rod Lens System, now the standard optical design for cystoscopes and other endoscopic telescopes. The first instrument was made only to inspect the bladder and take photographs and was not intended to be used for endoscopic surgery as the diameter was too large. Even with this improved optical system, which allowed as much as ten times the amount of light to be transmitted as through a conventional system, the illumination given by the 6-volt bulb at the end of the telescope was not sufficient for satisfactory photographs to be taken. As fibre-optics were not then available, a special filament bulb which could be used for both viewing and photography, and which could be fitted to the end of the telescope, was designed. The filament was normally lit by a 6-volt supply, but when photography was required, was over-run to 24 volts. Photographs were taken by attaching a small camera to the eyepiece of the telescope. The shutter mechanism of the camera was integrated with the transformer, which was used to increase the voltage from 6 to 24, so that when the shutter mechanism was released, there was an automatic delay of 1/20th of a second so that the light in the bladder could reach maximum intensity before the shutter opened. Figures 4.1 and 4.3 show this photographic equipment, which consists of a telescope, transformer and a camera. Figure 4.4 shows a sample of a photograph taken at that time with the telescope and reveals a quality which compares favourably with that produced today. The film used was super-anschochrome, 400 ASA. The next development was by Woolf, who produced a photoendoscope in the early 1960s (Fig. 4.5). This consisted of a sheath with a small lamp and a special optical system with a 110° field of view in air, equal to about 76° in water, and a miniature electronic flash system fitted in the terminal part of the telescope. To initiate the flash, only conventional camera contacts

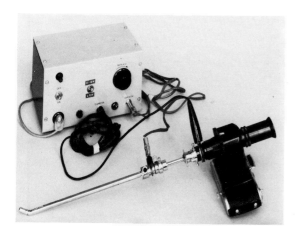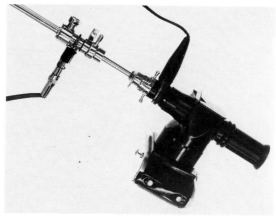

Figs. 4.1 and 4.2   Original Hopkins photographic instrument.

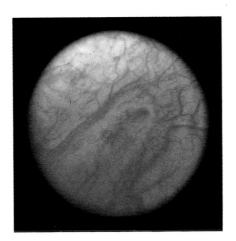

Fig. 4.4
Photograph of ureteric orifice taken
with the instrument.

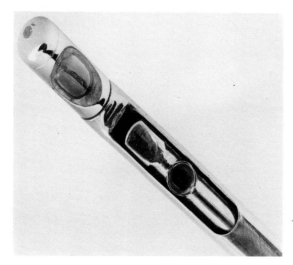

Fig. 4.3   Bulb attached to the end of the original Hopkins' Rod Lens Telescope.

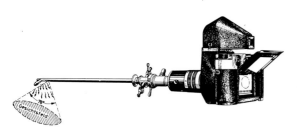

Fig. 4.5   Instrument designed by Woolf, courtesy of F. K. Schatteuer, Editor, Bauer's Cystoscopic Diagnosis.

were necessary and so any orthodox camera could be used. The power pack, which supplied the electronic flash, was used also to incorporate a light source for the low voltage lamp at the end of the sheath. Pictures of excellent detail were taken with this instrument, but the colour rendering was unacceptable, owing to the poor transmission of the blue end of the spectrum by the optical system in the telescope leaving a predominantly red-orange picture. The same criticisms applied to the colour produced by the bulb at the end of the telescope, which because of its size, produced an orange coloured picture inadequately illuminated. There was however, considerable improvement in both respects when the filament was over-run. At that time the problems waiting to be solved were, the restricting size of the instrument, excess heat inside the bladder and the danger of breakage. The discovery of fibre-optics meant that an external light source of high luminance could be used and the light transmitted through a flexible fibre cable to the telescope and then down the telescope to the distal end. This was a major step forward in the design of the modern cystoscope and allowed larger areas of the bladder to be inspected

with improved illumination due to the increased angle of field. Despite the excellent design of the new rod-lens telescope and the intense illumination from an external light source, photography of the bladder was unsuccessful with the routine instruments used in urological practice, because not enough light could be conveyed through an instrument which had an outside diameter of only 4 mm, as endoscopic surgery demands the use of operative instruments as well as the telescope within the lumen of the sheath. The size of the telescope is standardised to a maximum of 4 mm diameter. Consequently as the diameter of the lens system itself is 2·7 mm there is a limit to the number of glass fibres that can be mounted in the space between the lenses and the surrounding tube. These dimensions determine that however good the lens system is in transmitting the image the quality of photography will be governed by the amount of light that can be conveyed through the glass fibres to the object.

Factors affecting the use of telescopes in photography

Intensity of illumination in endoscopic image

The effective source of the illumination is the end of the fibre bundle, which is flush with the distal end of the endoscope. The intensity of illumination on the object is governed by the inverse square law which states that if the object distance is doubled to maintain the same intensity of illumination, the object plane would require a light source of 4 times the power. It is obvious, therefore, that as the distance from the bladder to the instrument is varied the intensity of the illumination on the bladder wall will follow this law. Consequently, the amount of light collected and conveyed to the surgeon's eye by the endoscope, will be reduced by a factor of 4 if he increases the distance to the bladder wall by a factor of 2. This phenomenon is experienced in every day practice as the farther the telescope is withdrawn from the bladder wall the darker the image becomes.

Focal length of camera lens

The radius of the image on any film is directly dependent on the focal length of the camera lens, hence the area depends on the square of the focal length. Since the total amount of light is constant, once the object distance is fixed, the intensity of illumination on the film plane can be increased by a factor of 4 by halving the focal length of the camera lens. It is because, reducing the focal length of the camera reduces the size of the image on the film plane, that, in practice, the operator tries to use the longest focal length consistent with a good picture.

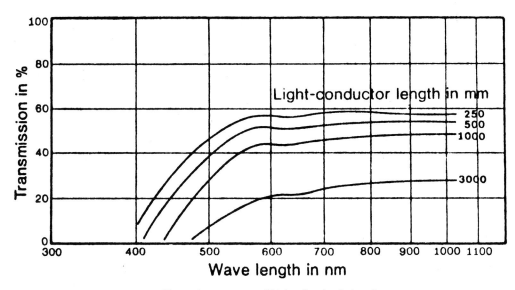

Fig. 4.6 Absorption spectrum of high refractive index glass.

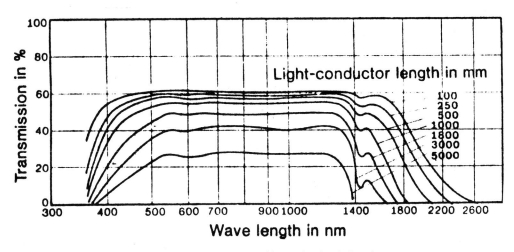

Fig. 4.7 Absorption spectrum of low refractive index glass.

The illumination system related to photography

Type of glass

The angle of view of the optical system in the modern telescope is designed to be 70° in water. If this area is to be uniformly illuminated, the core glass must have a high refractive index, but this type of glass has one great drawback, it absorbs about 90 per cent of the blue light over a length of two metres (Fig. 4.6). To overcome this complication the glass in the fibre cable is made of a glass of lower refractive index, which has a satisfactory transmission of the blue end of the spectrum (Fig. 4.7), but because it has a lower refractive index will not produce an illuminating core angle of 70° in water. To counter-act this, the fibres in the telescope are made of a glass of a refractive index of approximately 1·75 and the fibre cable of lower refractive index is coned down in order to adapt the beam of light in the fibre cable to the fibres in the telescope (Fig. 4.8). This arrangement is a compromise to enable the maximum amount of blue light to reach the bladder.

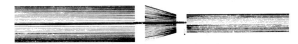

Fig. 4.8 Arrangement of adapting fibres in fibre cable to fibres in telescope.

D

Fibre optics

The discovery of fibre optics and its application to endoscopic medicine was the second outstanding physics discovery which improved the performance of endoscopic instruments and which consequently was of inestimable value to countless numbers of patients.

The fibre bundles consist of about 1000 glass fibres of between 70–100μ diameter bonded at the ends by an epoxy resin. Each of these fibres is covered by another glass, fused to the surface of the basic core glass, called the cladding. The function of the cladding is to prevent the escape of light from the surface of the core glass, when the light is transmitted down the fibre and to prevent the core glass becoming scratched and dirty, which would then lead to light leakage. As there are about 10,000 internal reflections when light passes along a 2 metre length of glass fibre, it can be appreciated that the reflection coefficient must be extremely high if an unacceptable amount of light is not going to be lost.

Loss of light during transmission from the source to the object

Figure 4.9 shows the system from the light source to the telescope and the various places where light is lost.

These are the six glass surfaces in the condenser system, light absorption in the fibre bundle, the loss of the packing fraction and at each end of the glass-air interface, and the connection with the cone in the telescope pillar together with more absorption in the glass fibre bundle in the telescope. When all these are multiplied together only about 11 per cent of light from the light source is useful. It has been suggested that, it would be better if there were an integral fibre bundle from the end of the telescope to the light source. If this method were adopted, a high refractive index glass must be used. This arrangement increases the light transmission to about 20 per cent, but the increased absorption of the blue end of the spectrum will make the picture a predominantly orange-red colour, one which is quite unacceptable for photography, especially with the Tungsten Halogen lamp, which is inadequate in power and has only a small percentage of its energy emission at the blue end of the spectrum (Fig. 4.10).

Problems of photography

The problem of photography is to transmit enough light to the object to take photographs of satisfactory colour and definition. The basic unchangeable essentials are a telescope of fixed size packed with as many fibres

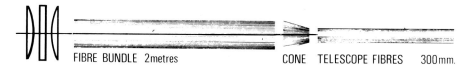

FIBRE BUNDLE 2 metres   CONE   TELESCOPE FIBRES   300 mm.

Fig. 4.9   Places where light is lost in system conveying light from external source to the end of the telescope.

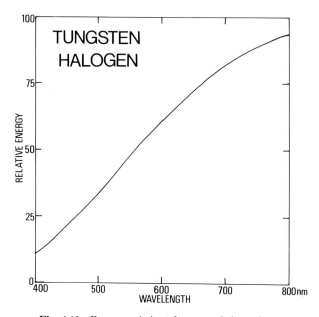

Fig. 4.10   Energy emission of tungsten halogen lamp.

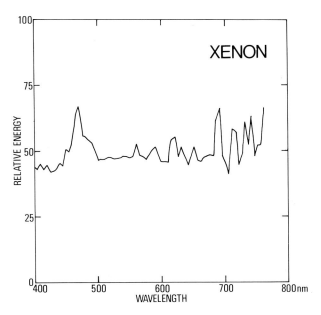

Fig. 4.11   Energy emission of xenon arc.

as can be fitted in the space available and which contains an optical system of advanced design with triple anti-reflection coating of the lenses. The only way to increase the light transmitted is to choose a source of light of the highest luminance. The standard lamp is the Tungsten Halogen lamp, which is unsatisfactory. The Xenon arc is the alternative as this gives from three to six times the luminance of the Tungsten Halogen and has an even spectral power distribution throughout the visible spectrum (Fig. 4.11). However, even the 500W Xenon arc does not provide sufficient light for accurate colour photography when it is conveyed through a 2-metre fibre bundle. The next choice is to attach the external light source to the pillar of the telescope so removing the main cause of the light loss absorption, as the light does not need to pass down a fibre bundle. The most satisfactory source for this purpose is a small Xenon U tube electronic flash unit, which has an even spectral power emission, similar to the Xenon arc, and which can be discharged as 500 joules, giving a much higher luminance than it is possible to obtain from the 500W Xenon arc. Units have been designed for this purpose, but even these will only allow satisfactory pictures to be taken if a high speed Ectochrome film is used and the focal length of the camera lens not more than 70 mm. The existing flash units have the added disadvantage that the light from the conventional source for viewing the bladder passes through the flash tube which reduces the intensity to such an extent that focussing of the object, to achieve accurate interpretation, is at best difficult and often impossible. To overcome this problem,

the medical optics unit at Reading has designed a flash unit, which gives greater illumination of the object in normal viewing, and thus allows more accurate focussing of the image in the camera. The light for viewing is transmitted through a prism to the pillar of the telescope and so does not have to pass through the flash tube for normal viewing of the bladder. When

FLASH UNIT MK II
optical layout – end view

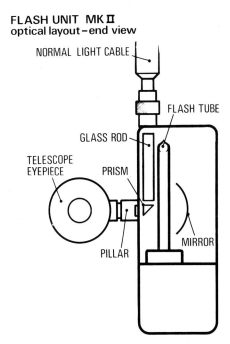

Fig. 4.12   End view of flash unit with moveable prism.

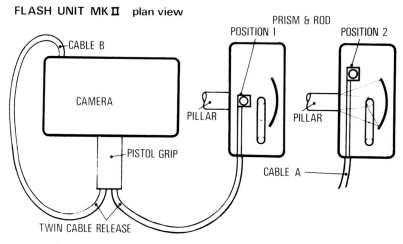

Fig. 4.13   Flash unit with prism in position for flash transmission.

the flash is operated for photography, the prism is automatically moved away. Figure 4.12 shows the end view of this unit. The light from the normal cable is carried to the pillar through a glass rod and prism. The triggering system of the camera contains two elements, one to release the shutter and the other to move away the rod and prism to allow the flash to be imaged onto the pillar by the rear concave mirror. As soon as the trigger is pressed, the cable moves the prism and rod from position 1 to 2 (Fig. 4.13). Cable B operates the camera shutter and flash supply, which is synchronously released when position 2 is reached (Fig. 4.13). Even this unit will only permit satisfactory photography using a focal length of 80 mm at a distance of not more than 20 mm from the bladder wall. These conditions are not acceptable for routine use, because of the inadequate diameter on the bladder covered by the given field size at the distance of 20 mm. There seemed therefore no alternative but to increase the size of the telescope. If the telescope diameter were increased to 5 mm and the optical system remained unchanged in diameter, 4 times the number of fibres could be fitted into the telescope, and this would allow 4 times the amount of light to be transmitted to the bladder. With this change and the new flash unit it should be possible to take satisfactory colour pictures at a focal length of 90 to 100, 25–30 mm from the bladder wall. In a previous chapter, the principle of interchangeability and standardisation of endoscopic instruments has been stressed. The adoption of two large telescopes of 30° and 70° respectively, for inspection and photography would not contradict this principle, as, although the larger telescopes would be essential for photography they could also be used for laparoscopy, choledo-

choscopy and nephroscopy. Two options would be open; either to have standard 70° and 30° telescopes, each of 4 mm diameter, as at present, and keep the 5 mm diameter for photography only, or else to have the 30° and 70° telescopes of 5 mm diameter telescopes for inspection and photography and keep the standard 30° telescope for endoscopic surgery. Using the larger telescope would increase the amount of light transmitted and would allow much greater freedom in the choice of films, and so further improve the colour reproduction in the picture.

It is important, that if photography is to become a standard part of endoscopic procedures, the technique must be simple, readily available, easy to carry out and relatively inexpensive. Until recently, the only way to take satisfactory endoscopic photographs was to attach the flash unit to the pillar of the telescope and the camera to the eyepiece. With this technique, it was time consuming, and focussing of the object through the camera was cumbersome and difficult, as well as being an unsterile procedure. When a new articulated lens dual viewing aid (DVA) became available the camera could be attached to the eyepiece of the dual viewing aid and pictures taken by an assistant. This, however, meant that the camera, unless it had been carefully calibrated beforehand had to be focussed by the assistant. This method, again, was time consuming and cumbersome and required the assistant to have some knowledge of photography. The next stage will be to design a small, cheap, light, automatic-loading camera using a simple objective lens of fixed focal length and giving satisfactory picture resolution. This camera would be attached to the DVA and photographs could then be taken by any assistant, who would simply release the shutter on the request of the operator, the focussing of the object being carried out by the endoscopist himself. It is to be hoped that before long such a photographic 'package', consisting of either a 70° or 30°, 5 mm diameter telescope, a simple flash unit, a DVA and a cheap camera will become part of every endoscopist's kit.

The photographs in this book were taken through the System 80, either the 30° or the 70°, telescope using the flash unit as described, with a high speed Ectochrome film. The focal length of the camera was kept constant at 70 mm.

5. Sterilisation of endoscopic instruments

Organisms are all around us. Most of them are harmless, a few may even be useful, others however, may be dangerous and produce serious disease. Control of organisms has absorbed the time of bacteriologists for over a hundred years, and the problem of sterilising what appears to be unsterilisable will remain with us and test our skill and ingenuity for many years to come. Before embarking on discussion of the various methods, it is essential to appreciate the precise understanding of three terms.

Sterilisation
This implies the complete destruction of all organisms, spores and viruses.

Disinfection
The destruction of harmful organisms but does not include the killing of bacterial spores.

Antisepsis
The destruction of organisms, not bacterial spores, which occur on living tissue.

Sterility is a vital part of modern medicine. Every effort must be made to keep away organisms from areas of the human body, where they can cause serious disease. Consequently, any instruments or dressings which are used in the investigation or treatment of surgical conditions must always be sterile.

Organisms vary in their resistance to sterilisation and this variant must be appreciated. The most sensitive are the vegetive organisms, more resistant are the acid first organisms such as the myco-tuberculosis and those that show the highest degree of resistance are spore forming organisms such as *clostridium.*

Heat is the most efficient way of killing organisms and the ideal method is steam under pressure. In the modern high vacuum autoclave vegetative organisms, spores and viruses will be killed within a few minutes and the whole cycle, starting with unsterile material and ending with clear sterile instruments ready for use, is completed in from 15 to 30 minutes. Unfortunately, this ideal method is not universally acceptable in the discipline of urology as many articles are too big, and others such as electric circuits and plastics cannot endure the intense heat, pressure or moisture. The problem, then, is to find alternative methods which will sterilise as efficiently as steam, and yet, leave delicate instruments undamaged. Sterility is a high ideal, but one which cannot always be achieved in urological practice, and in these circumstances it is suggested that they can be relaxed and disinfection accepted.

Disinfection is a less exact term than sterilisation and therefore, a less definitive process. It only implies freedom from infection and makes objects safe to handle. There are many situations and occasions in hospital practice, where bacterial spores do not create a problem and in these situations sterilisation is not vital—disinfection is. Although disinfection is acceptable in certain aspects of urological practice, when applied to urological instruments it is important that satisfactory cleaning of the instruments should be undertaken before the disinfection process is instituted, as adequate cleaning removes a high proportion of organisms including spores.

A satisfactory technique, used in the author's practice, is to soak the sheaths and the telescopes in an enzyme solution for five minutes. They are then removed, and the telescopes and the outsides of the sheaths are sponged with distilled water. The inside of the sheath is cleaned with an endotracheal brush large enough to give good contact with the sides of the lumen. The instruments are then ready for sterilisation or disinfection.

CHEMICAL DISINFECTANTS

The development and promotion of chemical disinfectants is a competitive business and the medical profession is constantly being visited by representatives attempting to persuade them that first of all disinfectants are essential and secondly that the one in which they are particularly interested is far superior to all others on the market. Persistent persuasion produces the danger of creating a belief that the use of a particular disinfectant fluid removes the risk of contamination by organisms. It is mandatory, therefore, to use an objective approach in ascertaining the potential of disinfectant fluids and to condemn those that have no value. What is certain, is that there is no miracle fluid and equally certain, that there never will be. In making an objective assessment various chemical groups must be considered and they should fulfil the following criteria:

1. They should be rapid acting, simple and safe.
2. They should kill bacteria as well as spores.
3. They should be able to act in the presence of serum or other organic matter.
4. They should be of low toxicity in small concentrations.
5. They must not react with materials and produce toxic effects.

Even if all these criteria are fulfilled, any method must always be considered suspect as it is impossible to guarantee contact between the organism and the disinfectant for the desired length of time.

Table 5.1 shows the antibacterial activity of various chemical compounds. These figures are based on the optimum conditions, which are not always reached. When considering activity it should be appreciated that the conditions are rarely optimum and therefore, a much greater time in contact with the organisms may be required and this should be allowed for. For any disinfectant fluid to be effective it must come in contact with bacteria and be absorbed by them. It is, therefore, essential that any cleaning of instruments should be carried out prior to immersion in solution. If contamination is severe, instruments can first be left in a solution to destroy surface organisms then removed, cleaned and re-immersed for a further period of time, to achieve the maximum disinfection.

To obtain the best results from disinfecting fluids, it is advisable to comply with the instructions of the manufacturer and it is especially important that the time factor should be taken into account. All disinfectants take time to act and this time factor varies with each disinfectant. Most disinfectants will produce satisfactory control of organisms within half an hour, but this is by no means universal. What is certain, is that the longer the immersion or the longer the organism is in contact with the disinfectant the more effective is its action.

This time factor applies up to 30 hours or longer, but most disinfectants deteriorate over a period of time and consequently solutions should be freshly prepared. In cases of B. proteus, which have been reported growing in hibitane solutions, this may well be due to the solution being too old and beginning to deteriorate and in these circumstances, bacteria, which may survive, can begin to multiply and be a source of cross infection.

It is an excellent practice that a solution is replaced daily and a higher concentration than that which is required should be used. It is also important that the containers in which the solution is placed be heat sterilised by a high vacuum autoclave prior to use. Chemical disinfectants are inactivated by materials such as soap, blood, pus, vomit and faeces and some food stuffs especially milk. Man-made material such as nylon and polyurethane has been shown to reduce the activity of disinfectants and should not be used as receptacles in which instruments are placed. If chemical disinfectants are decided to be used it is essential to aim for optimum conditions, i.e.

1. Cleansing of the instruments.
2. A container that does not cause deterioration of the antiseptic.
3. Replacement of the antiseptic every twenty-four hours with a higher concentration of the antiseptic than is required.
4. Contact with the organism for as long a period as possible.

Chemical disinfectants should only be considered when heat is impossible as all groups have disadvantages. There are only three groups that have any value in urological practice. The alcohols, the aldehydes, and chlorhexidine.

The alcohols

Alcohol is a satisfactory substance to use for the dis-

Table 5.1 Activity of some chemical compounds against various organisms. Published data

Organism	Test period	Cidex	Hibitane	Formaldehyde alcoholic sol.	Alcohol
Staphylococcus aureus	$\frac{1}{2}$ min	kills	kills	kills	no kills
Haemolytic streptococcus	$\frac{1}{2}$ min	kills	kills	kills	kills
E. coli	$\frac{1}{2}$ min	kills	kills	kills	kills
Pseudomonas aeroginosa	2 min	kills	kills	kills	kills
Proteus vulgaris	$\frac{1}{2}$ min	kills	kills	kills	kills
Myco-tuberulosis	10 min	kills	no kill	kills	kills
Coxsa coxsackie	10 min	kills	no activity	kills	no kill
Echo 6 ⎫ virucidal	10 min	kills	no activity	kills	no kill
B. subtilis ⎭ activity	3 hrs	kills	no kill	kills	no kill
Cl. tetani ⎫ sporicidal	3 hrs	kills	no kill	kills	no kill
Cl. welchii ⎭ activity	3 hrs	kills	no kill	kills	no kill

infection of skin, thermometers or other simple instruments. It is unsuitable for use with any organic material, as it penetrates poorly, and is of little value in the presence of organic material, because of this inadequate penetration. It should not be used undiluted, the concentration between 70° and 90° is satisfactory. It is rarely used alone, but with iodine or chlorhexidine added, has considerable use in the disinfection of urological instruments.

Aldehydes

The aldehydes can be a most effective disinfectant under optimum conditions but as these are rarely obtained they have serious disadvantages. Formaldehyde is used as a gas or in a 40 per cent solution as formalin. Both cause intense irritation to the mucous membranes especially of the eyes, where lacrimation is frequent and severe. Its penetration of fabrics is poor and its use now has very little place in modern urological practice. However, gluteraldehyde, an analogue of the aldehydes, is a much more active substance and comes near to the satisfactory disinfectant. It is the buffered dialdehyde solution which has two active carbonyl groups. These groups react with protein and prevent the normal biochemical processes required for growth of bacteria. It is slightly acid, is highly soluble in water, has diminished activity in the acid state, is not sporicidal, is unaffected by the presence of up to 20 per cent serum and its toxicity for living cells is low. However, when buffered to between pH 7·5 and 8·5 in concentrations of 2 per cent the solution is active against vegetative organisms, mycotuberculosis, viruses, fungi and spores. It can kill all common organisms within five minutes, myco-tuberculosis within ten, and fungacidal spores also within five. Unfortunately, it took up to three hours to kill vegetative spores, hence the limitations in its use for sterilisation purposes. Once activated, the solution remains active for about two weeks, but after this time, its activity diminishes because of oxidation products. For the best results, it should be used within one week of activation. In addition, to its cidal properties it had other physical advantages. It has no effect on cement or chemical substances used in the manufacture of optical systems, so that endoscopic instruments may be left for many hours in a solution of gluteraldehyde without producing any adverse effects.

Being an aqueous solution it rinses easily, and provided that the rinsing is complete, only a very small quantity remains, and, in one experiment, less than eight parts per million was found to be left on a rubber tube. It is non-corosive, does not effect sharp surfaces or cause blunting of needles, does not coagulate blood or other protein material and consequently does not add to the problem of cleaning instruments between cases. Occasionally, corosion poses an electrolytic type of problem, if two or more dissimilar metals are present in the same solution. For example, if aluminium and steel instruments are to be disinfected with gluteraldehyde, each should be immersed in a separate tray. It is important that if stainless steel trays are used plastic mats should be placed in the bottom to prevent metal to metal contact.

Toxic effect

Inhalation of formaldehyde vapour causes intense irritation in the respiratory tract and may give rise to bronchitis. Sensitisation reactions occur from the use of formaldehyde on the skin. Gluteraldehyde is less irritant to skin and mucous membranes than formaldehyde, but it may cause sensitisation and repeated contact with the skin should be avoided. Two out of 40 nursing staff exposed to gluteraldehyde in the theatre developed a contact dermatitis confirmed by the patch testing. The writer is unable to use instruments which have been soaked in gluteraldehyde as they can cause conjunctivitis, periorbital inflammation and oedema.

Chlorhexidine

Chlorhexidine is an antiseptic active against a wide spectrum of pathogens retaining its activity in high dilutions. Its mode of action is a reaction with the negatively charged group of cells on the surface of organisms. Its effect depends on the amount of chlorhexidine absorbed. High concentrations cause rapid bacteriocidal action. Eventually, the plasma of the cell becomes coagulated and cellular proteins are precipitated. It is, however, inactivated in the presence of pus and serum and against myco-tuberculosis it is only bacteriocidal in 70 per cent of alcohol solution. It is only sporicidal in high temperatures and cannot be considered a sporicidal agent. It is effective over a wide range of pH, but its most effective area is 7·2. It is adversely affected by soap and detergents, hence thorough cleaning of instruments is important before immersion. If used for sterilising instruments either 0·5 or 1 per cent solution in 70 per cent of alcohol is the best combination. In these concentrations it will kill staphylococcals, E. coli, B. proteus and pseudomonas within ten minutes of contact time. If employed for sterilising instruments, users must be aware that some cements used in telescopic construction may be damaged. With modern cements this is unlikely, but even so occasional leakage occurs, especially after a prolonged period of time. What is most important is, that once this method of sterilisation has been employed, transfer to heat sterilisation is absolutely contra-indicated as one followed by the other, would almost certainly mean the softening of the cement and an inevitable leak in the optical system. When used, hibitane should be prepared fresh daily and discarded after use.

Sporicidal activity of chemical disinfectants

The importance of spores in urinary tract infection and endoscopic surgery is small. However, if outbreaks are to be prevented spores should be killed whenever possible. Chemical disinfectants are not reliable if complete sterilisation is required. Some, such as gluteraldehyde, show sporicidal activity but the time is prolonged and it is a very poor substitute for heat sterilisation. Nevertheless, there are times when heat sterilisation is not practical and in these cases the use of disinfectants may have to be employed and only two solutions which should be considered in this context are gluteraldehyde and chlorhexidine.

Gluteraldehyde failed all tests with the watery spores, but with the alcoholic spores cidex killed during the first three days of activation but failed each of the following ten days (Kelsey, 1974). Gluteraldehyde was only really effective on the day of activation and is not recommended to be used in any other way, when the sporicidal effect is desired. Gluteraldehyde is a poor sporicide, consequently, it should only be used for the disinfection of instruments between cases. At the end of the day, some other method should be employed so that complete sterilisation can be achieved. Hibitane completely failed with the concentration of 10 per cent up to three hours of contact. Failures occurred with both alcoholic and watery spores. Therefore, if it is used, it must be realised that the combination has no sporicidal activity.

Ethylene oxide

Ethylene oxide has been used extensively to sterilise heat sensitive materials, such as plastic and in ideal circumstances can be considered a sterilising agent. It penetrates well and does not damage a wide spectrum of materials, is active against all organisms including viruses and spores and can be used under low temperature. The gas, however, is toxic, inflammable, and careful monitoring of its concentration, temperature and humidity is obligatory. Consequently, the apparatus is complex, expensive, requires skilled personnel and constant microbiological supervision. Furthermore, long post-sterilisation periods which are neither convenient nor practical in the normal hospital running are required to ensure that all the toxic gases are dispersed. Specialised monitoring may on occasions take up to seven or ten days, which, in itself, bars its use from a normal urological practice. It is also important to ensure that the residual ethylene oxide levels, on the item sterilised, are low enough to cause no toxic or irritant effect. Therefore, a period of up to twenty-four hours is essential so that all the gas can be evacuated and a special store for this purpose is required. Acceptable levels of residual gas are low and sophisticated methods are required for their detection, and

although this may not be a problem with telescopes as the metal is unlikely to absorb significant levels of Ethylene Oxide, it is uneconomic to consider installing expensive equipment only to sterilise metal instruments. Humidity and temperature are vital conditions of the sterilisation process with ethylene oxide and a humidity of 20–40 per cent and a temperature of approximately 80° is required for its effective action. It forms an explosive mixture with air and 12 per cent of carbon dioxide mixture is added to the air to reduce its explosive potential. It is soluble in water, rubber, certain plastics and has excellent penetration, but it is effected by dirt and serum and cannot be considered a reliable method when these substances are present. To be effective, a high standard of cleaning is required. In all methods of disinfection, the cleansing process is most important as it can remove a large percentage of all organisms, including any bacterial spores present. The value of cleaning as a disinfectant in its own right or combined with some other method of disinfection cannot be over emphasised. To be used effectively, therefore, ethylene oxide requires frequent microbiological monitoring as well as facilities for detecting residual ethylene oxide. If this method of disinfection is employed in a unit, the number of urological instruments must be above average, both to compensate for the time required for sterilisation of the instruments, and the long periods in which the instruments are out of use, so as not to disrupt an established clinical practice. As all these requirements are most unlikely to be met in most hospitals, it is doubtful, whether ethylene oxide has any place in routine sterilisation of urological instruments.

HEAT STERILISATION

Heat is the cheapest and most effective method of sterilisation and disinfection, and should be used whenever possible. There are two methods:

Dry heat sterilisation

Microbes are killed by this method by oxidation. Sealed containers are used, but a relatively long exposure time is needed if all the spores have to be killed. The recommended temperatures are shown in Table 5.2. With this method of sterilisation it is difficult to ensure that all items that are being sterilised, are held at the required temperature for the necessary time and special apparatus and techniques are required. It is the method of choice, for sterilising syringes and can be used for metal instruments. However, now that high vacuum autoclaves do not effect cutting edges and are becoming more efficient, this method has few applications and is becoming obsolete because of

E

Table 5.2   Times of temperatures for heat sterilisation

Method	Temperature °C	Time mins.
Autoclave	121	15
	126	10
	134	3
	150	Almost instantaneous
Oven	160	45
	170	18
	180	$7\frac{1}{2}$
	190	$1\frac{1}{2}$

the sophisticated monitoring apparatus that is required. It has no place in a modern urological unit.

Wet heat sterilisation

Microbes are killed by wet heat by the denaturation of proteins. The process is rapid, the exposure time is short and the times recommended by the Medical Research Council for sterilisation by exposure to steam are shown in Table 5.2. Most modern sterilisers are of the high vacuum type. The operation is complex and careful monitoring is essential to ensure that there are no variations from heat and temperature, as these would invalidate the sterilising process. British Standard Specification now insists on the use of automatic monitoring devices, which do not permit the procedure to take place, unless all the required conditions have been satisfied. What then is the use of such an instrument in urological practice? Any article which can be sterilised by moist heat using a high vacuum machine and which can be repeatedly sterilised without deterioration should be sterilised in this way. Such items are resecting and operating sheaths, resectoscope mechanisms, biopsy forceps, catheter deflectors, lithotrites and small parts such as extension pieces, catheter guides and taps. If such a method of sterilisation is available particularly with the modern high speed autoclave, the number of these articles that would be required by a particular unit will be reduced, as they can be sterilised between cases of a normal endoscopy session.

Boiling water

Boiling water cannot be used to sterilise. It will not kill spores and is now an obsolete way of attempting sterilisation or disinfection and should never be used.

Pasteurisation

The name is dedicated to Louis Pasteur who discovered that mild heating prevented the disintegration of wine by removing unnecessary organisms. This method was then applied to prevent the souring of milk. In hospital practice, instruments have been designed to use, either hot water or steam for pasteurisation. The minimum temperature recommended is 65° for 10 minutes in the presence of moisture. At higher temperatures shorter times may be satisfactory and for instruments 10 minutes between 65° and 75° should be satisfactory. Such times are holding times and an extra period has to be allowed for the apparatus to reach the required temperature. Whilst pasteurisation will kill most organisms, viruses, fungi, non-sporing bacteria including myco-tuberculosis and the spore formers whilst they are in active phase, it must be realised that pasteurisation is not a sterilisation process and will not kill bacterial spores.

Hot water pasteurisers

A purpose built hot water pasteuriser is convenient for the disinfection of instruments such as cystoscopes where disinfection is acceptable. Most of these that are used have a pre-set timer and the temperature is raised to the required level and kept for the holding period of 10 minutes. This period is monitored and the instrument is switched off automatically at the end of the agreed time. Most instruments have a device whereby if the lid is accidentally opened the machine is switched off, the timer is reset and a further 10 minute cycle is commenced. The problem about pasteurisers is the temperature control and the difficulty of keeping the temperature within the required tolerance because if the temperature rises above a certain level then damage to delicate instruments will occur. Pasteurisation can be carried out by steam through purpose-built instruments. The articles are exposed to temperatures of 80°C for 5 minutes or 70°C for 15 minutes, both of which are adequate for disinfection but with the availability of efficient low pressure steam autoclaves this method of disinfection is becoming obsolete.

Low pressure steam

Pioneer work on low pressure steam autoclaves was carried out by Mitchell and Alder (1963). The result of this work is now assuming great importance in view of the sophisticated design of modern endoscopic telescopes. These telescopes are delicate and extremely expensive. As yet no satisfactory means has been found whereby such instruments can be sterilised in high pressure steam autoclaves without damage to the lenses or to the cement, which is used to seal the instrument. Mitchell and Alder have demonstrated conclusively that low pressure steam can be used in Urological Units not only to sterilise instruments after sessions have been completed but also to disinfect instruments which are being employed in endoscopic sessions thus ensuring a rapid turnover. This means that telescopes can be used repeatedly during an endoscopy session, thus obviating the necessity of having large numbers of instruments, which would be the only alternative if the instruments could not be disinfected immediately after use, and yet, still provide an adequate service.

The concept of sterlisation and disinfection of modern endoscopes is changing and it is important that one should endeavour to sterilise or disinfect instruments by heat between each case. It is reasonable to relax the standards to a certain degree especially as regards spores. This relaxation should be tempered to the work involved. It should not be considered a justification unless risks are minimal. Until recently, low pressure steam sterilisation or disinfection was not possible because there was no satisfactory instrument available. Recently, however, a new low pressure steam autoclave has been produced by Thackray called the miniclave (Figs. 5.1 & 5.2).

The miniclave is a self-contained unit which requires only a 15 amp power source. It incorporates reservoirs for water and formalin which are easy to fill, generates its own steam and has a discharge tank. The chamber measures $10'' \times 18''$ and has a capacity of 3 to 4 cysto-

scopic sets packed in boxes. The sterilising temperatures are 73° and/or −2° and a safety cut-out operates if the temperature exceeds 80°C. Sterilising pressure is 427–513 ml of mercury and the cycle time is approximately 60 minutes. The formalin cycles are set at 3 ml formalin injection and 20 minutes exposure but these can be varied according to requirements. There are six stages (Fig. 5.3).

1. The air is removed with steam pulses.
2. The formalin is then injected, the factory pre-set at 3 ml per cycle and variable according to the conditions, 0–18 ml being available.
3. Sterilisation time again variable pre-set 20 minutes for general use, but 4–210 minutes are available.
4. Elution steam pulses to wash out residual formalin.
5. Drying time again variable pre-set four minutes, changeable according to conditions.
6. Air admitted to the chamber through a bacterial filter.

The steam consumption varies according to the differential of the vacuum switch, but at all times 10 cycles per filling of the water reservoir can be obtained. The formalin consumption varies with the time settings from 3 ml at 0·4 seconds to 21 ml at 5 seconds. The cycle time is 33 minutes with a completely empty chamber, 38–40 minutes with a full chamber contained in a cardboard carton.

Sophisticated safety circuits ensure that the cycle cannot be started unless the door is closed and both the steam generator and chamber are at the correct temperature. When the miniclave is switched on, the steam generator and chamber begin to heat. Once the correct temperature has been reached and the door closed, the cycle can be commenced. The chamber is sealed by a sliding door using the Thackray autoclamp pressure sealing system, which prevents the door being operated until the chamber is at atmospheric pressure. This is a safety device which eliminates the necessity for mechanical locking mechanisms and reduces maintenance requirements. Other safety devices are incorporated, so that should the miniclave fail to maintain the correct sterilising conditions, an alarm will sound, the cycle will stop, air will be admitted to the chamber so that the load can be removed. A new cycle can only be commenced by passing the abortive cycle process and by use of the key-operated manual over-ride switch. A comprehensive test programme was arranged to confirm its efficiency and we are grateful to Dr. G. L. Gibson for the use of his data, namely test programmes designed to indicate the minimum exposure in terms of time, temperature and formaldehyde injection, which would reliably and consistently kill organisms and viruses.

Two different cycles were tested.

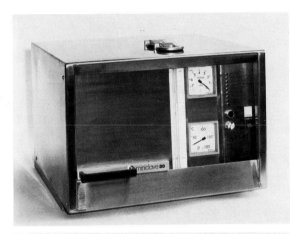

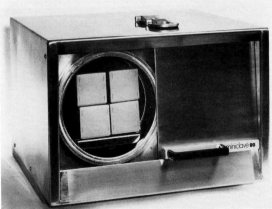

Figs. 5.1 and 5.2 The miniclave low pressure steam autoclave.

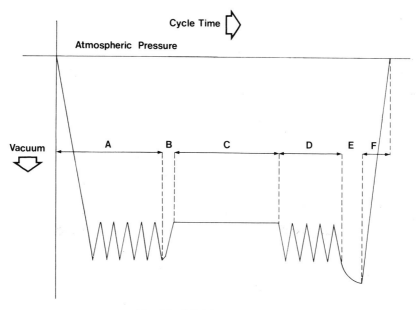

Fig. 5.3   Miniclave 80 cycle time.

1. A disinfectant cycle involving exposure to steam alone, with an exposure time of 20 minutes at 73°C. This cycle is intended to be used for processing cystoscopes between cases either at outpatient or inpatient sessions, thus ensuring a rapid turnover of a small number of instruments. The results are shown in Table 5.3.
2. The second cycle involved exposure to steam and formaldehyde and is intended to achieve sterilisation of endoscopes at the end of a session. Various tests were carried out.

(a) Table 5.4 shows the effect of formaldehyde and steam on B. stearothermophilus and demonstrates that the speed of action depends on the amount of formalin injected.
(b) Table 5.5 shows the result when the test organism was added to serum. In this test longer exposure to steam was required but there was less dependence on the concentration of formalin.
(c) Table 5.6 shows the results of serum impregnated test pieces placed within a cystoscope sheath and packed in boxes and demonstrates that effective killing of organisms and spores could be achieved by exposure to a combination of steam and formalin for two hours.

These results show that low pressure steam and formaldehyde is a satisfactory and reliable way of disinfecting and sterilising delicate instruments, which will not stand the full high pressure steam autoclave cycle. Exposure to steam alone, for 20 minutes dis-

Table 5.3   Disinfecting cycle. Exposure of organism to steam alone. (*Courtesy of :* G. L. Gibson)

	Time in minutes of steam exposure 73°C					
	1	2	5	10	20	30
Growth +	+ −	+ +	− −	− −	− −	− −
No Growth −						

Test Organisms—Staphylococcus aureus and Streptococcus faecalis

Table 5.4   Exposure of organism to steam and formaldehyde (*Courtesy of* G. L. Gibson)

Injection of Formalin in ml	Time in minutes of exposure to steam at 73 C				
	5	10	15	20	30
3	+ +	+ +	+ +	− −	− −
	+ +	+ +	− −	− −	− −
6	+ +	+ +	− −	− −	− −
	+ +	+ +	− −	− −	− −
9	+ +	− −	− −	− −	− −
	+ +	− −	− −	− −	− −
12	+ −	− −	− −	− −	− −
	− −	− −	− −	− −	− −
15	− −	− −	− −	− −	− −
	− −	− −	− −	− −	− −

+ = growth within 4 days   − = no growth within 4 days

Table 5.5 Serum soaked B. stearothermophilus spore strips. Syringe test piece. (*Courtesy of* G. L. Gibson)

Injection of Formalin in ml	Time in minutes of exposure to steam at 73°C						
	5	10	15	20	30	45	60
3	+ +	+ +	+ +	+ +	+ +	− −	− −
6	+ +	+ +	+ +	+ +	− +	− −	− −
9	+ +	+ +	+ +	+ +	− +	− −	− −
12	+ +	+ +	+ +	+ +	+ +	− −	− −
15	+ +	+ +	+ +	+ +	+ +	− −	− −

Tests in duplicate.
+ = growth after 4 days   − = no growth after 4 days

Table 5.6 Serum soaked B. stearothermophilus spore strip. Mitchell and Alder test piece. (*Courtesy of* G. L. Gibson)

Injection of Formaldehyde in ml	Time in minutes of exposure to steam at 73°C			
	60	90	120	180
1·5	+	+	−	−
3·0	+	+	+	−
6·0	+	−	+	−
9·0	+	−	−	−
12·0	+	+	−	−
15·0	+	+	−	−
18·0	+	−	−	−

+ = growth after 10 days   − = no growth after 10 days

infects instruments between cases at an endoscopic session and exposure to steam and formaldehyde for 2 hours will sterilise endoscopes after use and will keep them in a sterile condition until they are next required.

Suggested disinfection and sterilisation régime
All articles which will stand high pressure autoclave treatment should be sterilised by this method. The cycle takes between 5–20 minutes, and such articles of equipment can be sterilised between cases by this technique even if there is a long and continuous list of endoscopic examinations. Articles that will not stand high pressure autoclave, e.g. cystoscopic telescopes should be sterilised prior to use, by means of the low pressure steam, with formaldehyde. In between cases telescopes should be disinfected by means of the low pressure autoclave, without formaldehyde. At the end of the session the telescopes can be put through the much longer cycle of steam plus formaldehyde and stored for use at the next session. If low pressure steam autoclaves are not available, immersion in gluteraldehyde is the best method to disinfect the telescopes. However, if the operator is unable to use this substance because of hypersensitivity, then 0·5 to 1 per cent hibitane in 70 per cent spirit can be substituted. All techniques of disinfection involving hibitane and spirit should use this method continuously and under no consideration should this method of disinfection be followed by a low pressure steam autoclave as the combination will lead to damage of the lens cement resulting in leakage. As an alternative to hibitane, pasteurisation either by steam or hot water may be employed to disinfect telescopes.

It cannot be stressed too highly that with sophisticated and expensive endoscopic optical instruments, sterilisation by low pressure steam autoclaves is the best method available and should be used whenever possible.

REFERENCES

Alder, V. G., Gingell, J. C. and Mitchell, J. P. (1971). Disinfection of cystoscopes by subatmospheric steam and steam formaldehyde at 80°C. *British Medical Journal*, Sept. 18, **3**, 677–680.

Gibson, G. L. (1976). Processing urinary endoscopes in a low temperature steam and formaldehyde autoclave. In press.

Kelsey, J. C. (1970). Disinfectants for hospital use, an interim statement. *PHLS Monograph*, **2**, London, HMSO.

Kelsey, J. C. (1970). The myth of surgical sterility. *Lancet*, **Dec. 16,** 1301–1303.

Kelsey, J. C., MacKinnon, I. H. and Maurer, I. M. (1974). Sporicidal activity of hospital disinfectants. *Journal of Clinical Pathology*, **27**, 632–638.

6. Diathermy

Surgical diathermy is an essential part of endoscopic surgery and many surgeons are ignorant of and impervious to the possible damages which may be caused by the diathermy machine.

When an electric current passes through the body which acts as a resistance, heat is generated and this is the basis of surgical diathermy. There are two electrodes, the live and the indifferent. The live, producing cutting, coagulation or fulguration, the indifferent being the electrode which completes the circuit and through which the current is returned to the diathermy machine. The diathermy effect is produced through an arc struck between the live electrode and tissues. The temperature being in excess of 1000°C and as the density of the current is inversely proportional to the size of the electrode, the smaller the electrode the greater the heat and the more rapid the incision. The current from the live electrode disseminates through the patient's body and reaches the indifferent electrode which is large and is placed in intimate contact with the patient. As cutting and coagulation only take place at points of high current density, those conditions only achieved at the live electrode, there will be no effect at the point of contact with the indifferent electrode where the current density is too low, and provided basic safety standards are observed.

The machine

The principle of diathermy is based on the high frequency alternating currents which, passing through the body without stimulating, muscle and nerves, can be used either to coagulate or cut tissues depending on the heat generated at the point of contact. The heating effect is proportional to the strength of the current and size of the point of contact. The smaller the contact, the greater will be the heating effect.

The earliest diathermy machines produced a high frequency alternating current by means of a spark gap which provided bursts of a damped wave-form of about 500 waves at between 400–500 KHz occurring at irregular intervals. This type of wave-form gave satisfactory coagulation but even the maximum current was not powerful enough to allow satisfactory under water cutting.

The first valve machines were designed in 1926 and produced a typical sine-wave form in regular bursts of 50 cycles at a much higher frequency 2·5–3 MHz. This type of wave-form can strike a perfect arc causing disintegration of tissue with very little coagulation. A current produced in this way, was ideal for cutting but unsatisfactory for coagulation, unless turned down to minimal strength. Even though both types of wave-form can be made to coagulate and cut, it is much more efficient to provide a machine with both wave-forms, one to coagulate and the other to cut. It is vital for the urologist to have available both of these facilities. Modern machines provide 2 foot switches, one for cutting and the other for coagulation. These should be available for use during endoscopic resection, as and when they are required. Some manufacturers incorporate a 'blended current' in their machines. The word blended is inaccurate as it is not a composite current but a summation of the currents produced by the spark gap and valve circuits. It is questionable whether the use of this blended current is desirable or necessary, as not only is the total amount of current passing through the body increased but it is impossible to get the perfect blend, either one or the other predominates, giving an unsatisfactory end result. It seems far more logical to use each current independently, provided that the dual foot switch is always available. Until the last two to three years the combined valve and spark gap machine has been standard, but recently, transistorised diathermy machines, which can be designed to produce any wave form, have been developed. The main characteristic of diathermy machines is an ability to generate powerful high frequency currents and this can best be achieved by multiple transistors which in the output stage can generate 3–400 watts of power at a frequency of more than 400 KHz. This leads to difficulties in design, as equal power sharing in conjunction with variations of electrical conditions in patient's tissue and uncertain tolerances on components, is difficult to achieve.

Despite these problems the transistorised circuits have many advantages. They are smaller, and therefore, lighter machines can be constructed. They have a longer working life than valves and should not become impaired with age. The smaller working voltage should provide both improved safety and better control of power output, as it is easier to design control circuits at a transistor voltage of 50 volts than the valve

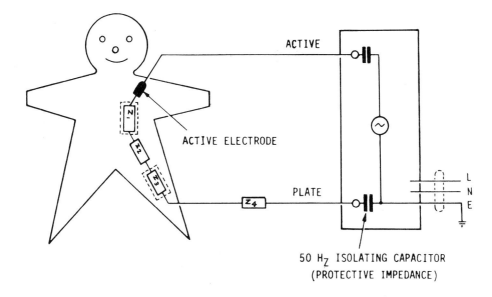

Z_1 represents the contact impedance between the active electrode and the patient, typically 500 ohms, mainly resistive.

Z_2 represents the impedance of the current path within the patient's body, typically 20 ohms, mainly resistive.

Z_3 represents the contact impedance between the plate electrode and the patient, typically 2 ohms, mainly resistive.

Z_4 represents the impedance of the plate cable, typically 30 ohms, mainly inductive.

Fig. 6.1 Typical arrangement of Diathermy connected to patient. D.H.S.S. Electro-Medical Equipment Data Sheet EU4.1 (by permission).

counterpart with more than 2000 volts. Furthermore, the transistorised circuits are potentially more efficient as they can be designed to generate any wave shape and the machines already produced are excellent. Lastly, the power circuit can be isolated by the use of a transformer so that there is no connection to earth. In this case, the live electrode is only connected to the individual through the indirect electrode and provided this is of adequate surface area, no burn can occur. This is an added safety measure and avoids the danger of an accidental burn should any part of the patient come in contact with return pathways other than the indifferent electrode. However, it must be realised, that transistors are much more electrically delicate devices than are valves and therefore are prone to disintegrate if overloaded. Hence they may give rise to maintenance problems after prolonged use, so that a period of time must elapse before their performance entitles them to supercede existing machines.

Figure 6.1 shows typical arrangement of diathermy connected to a patient.

There are three ways in which this high frequency current can be employed in surgery (Fig. 6.2).

Cutting
Cutting is achieved by employing a high frequency current between 2 and 5 mHz and using a very fine electrode or loop. The temperature produced is so high that cells disintegrate and the tissues separate as if they were cut by a knife. No coagulation takes place, but the tissue damage other than that close to the incision is minimal.

Coagulation
Coagulation occurs by a combination of cell destruction and the denaturing of proteins. Ideally the individual vessels should be identified, picked up with forceps and coagulated to limit the damage to surrounding tissue

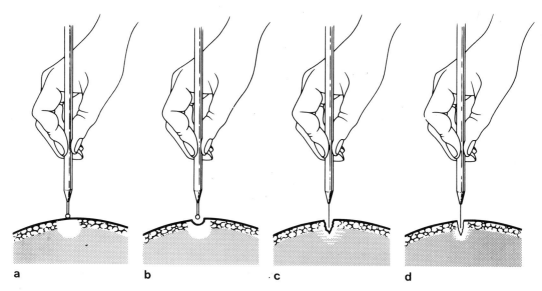

Fig. 6.2 Diagram of three effects of Diathermy. (a) Coagulation. (b) Fulguration. (c) Cutting (spark gap). (d) Cutting Valve. From Blandy, J. (1976) Urology (by permission).

which could delay healing and encourage infection. The smallest current compatible with effective coagulation should be used.

Fulguration

Fulguration occurs when a strong current is kept in contact with tissue long enough for charring to take place. It should never be used to obtain haemostasis as the destruction of tissue can only result in the formation of slough and slow healing. Its place in urology should be reserved for the destruction of bladder tumours where a wide area of cell destruction is required.

The indifferent electrode

The traditional indifferent electrode was made of lead so that it could be moulded easily to the contours of the body and give satisfactory contact. The size was calculated so that the heat generated with the maximum output of the machine was not sufficient to cause damage to the skin. They are normally made considerably larger than required to allow for poor contact and errors·in position. These electrodes have to be covered with layers of material soaked in an isotonic solution of sodium chloride to prevent water blisters. They are protected by a Mackintosh held in position by a tight bandage to preserve moisture, even so it may. be necessary during a long operation to remoisten the plate and it is advisable to inspect the indifferent electrode from time to time. The lead indifferent electrodes have stood the test of time and are efficient so long as they are kept constantly moist. However, in recent years, to a

large extent, they have been superceded by dry flexible metal electrodes. The dry flexible metal electrodes are of two types, the flexible metal and metal foil. They have many advantages being light, cheap and semi-disposable. Manufacturers recommend that they can be used up to ten times. They are bonded to a moulded rubber holder and can be sterilised if necessary by autoclaving. They have a surface area of over 200 cm^2 and the foil forms part of the monitoring control circuit, so that a failure in any part of the foil will operate the monitor warning system and render the diathermy inoperative. Preferably, they should be placed under the patient so that the patient's own weight guarantees good contact between the metal and skin, but they may also be strapped round the thigh. They should never be placed on the patient or over a bony area and once cracks or wrinkles have appeared they should be discarded. Hairy areas should be shaved before the plate is applied.

Position of the indifferent electrode

There is no one position that is ideal for all operations but the most efficient results are achieved if the plate is sited as close to the active electrode as possible. For endoscopic and abdominal surgery an excellent position is under the buttocks, but when it is being used in conjunction with surgery of the head and neck it should be placed on the arm, as it is inadvisable for the current pathways to cross the.heart. The plate should never be sited in an area of the body such as the calf so that current passing between the live and indifferent electrode has to cross a joint, as joints are very poor conductors.

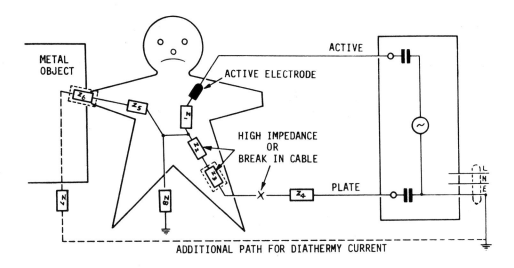

Z_5 represents impedance of alternative internal current path.

Z_6 represents contact impedance of patient to metal object.

Z_7 represents impedance to earth of metal object.

Z_8 represents the overall impedance (mainly capacitive) of the patient to earth.

BURN AT POINT OF CONTACT WITH METAL OBJECT

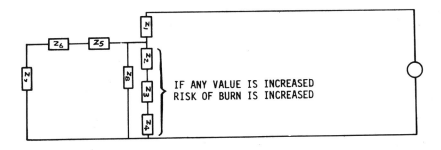

EQUIVALENT CIRCUIT OF FIGURE 5·3

Figs. 6.3 and 6.4 Burn at point of contact with metal object. D.H.S.S. Electro-Medical Equipment Data Sheet EU4.3 (by courtesy of A. K. Dobbie).

Diathermy in patients with cardiac pacemaker
Provided that due precautions are taken, there is no contra-indication for using diathermy resection on patients, who have been fitted with either internal or external cardiac pacemakers. Spinal or epidural anaesthesia is advisable and the operator must be certain that the diathermy is earthed adequately, that the current pathway does not cross the heart and that facilities must be on hand in case ventricular fibrillation develops. It is advisable to place the indifferent electrode under the buttocks. Care must be exercised in the use of ECG electrodes in the presence of diathermy. Burns occur very easily at the site of the needle electrode and it is important to make sure that the cable between the needle and the ECG machine is fitted with a 10,000 ohm resistance.

Hazards

Burns
The high current necessary to cut and coagulate tissue means that there is always a danger of causing serious burns to the patient. One of the commonest ways is the accidental operation of the foot pedal when the live electrode is not in use but is lying in contact with the patient or touching clamps or instruments, which are in contact with the patient. Burns caused in this way can be deep and take a long time to heal and may even require surgery.

Burns at the site of the plate electrode
The normal contact resistance between the plate electrode and the patient's skin is about 2 ohms. If due to part contact, the figure may be well above this mark, and the increased heat produced may cause a burn. Poor contact may be due to badly applied, bent or cracked plates, insufficient pressure at the site of application or in the case of a moist pad, failure to ensure that adequate moisture is retained. If the moist pad is used, it is better to site it on the thigh rather than under the buttocks as the pressure of the body on the plate is likely to cause rapid drying. Also it is more difficult to keep the plate moist in this position.

Burns between the patient and metal objects
Figure 6.3 and 6.4 demonstrate that the patient's body, under normal circumstances, has a resistance value of 50 ohms. If an alternative pathway occurs, the circuit prefers to take this pathway and a burn occurs at the point of contact between the patient's body and earth. This may be due to a fault in the indifferent electrode with a small area of contact between the electrode and the patient, and contact between the patient's body and an object, which is connected with earth, e.g. the metal part of an operating table. Coagulation can also occur if the internal current path is short, as the temperature and the tissue may rise sufficiently to result in unintended coagulation.

Explosion
No explosion is possible unless inflammatory anaesthetic gasses are present, and these play very little part in modern anaesthesia. Ether and cyclopropane are the only two that are likely to be employed and if it is necessary to use them, full precautions must be taken. Attempts have been made to produce spark proof diathermy machines but these are neither desirable or possible. The foot piece was another source of sparking, but now, the foot switch supply is restricted to 12 volts. Also the foot switches are fitted with water-tight rubber housings. To reduce static spark, diathermy machines have been fitted with an antistatic wheel. Despite all these safety precautions, it is wise to adopt the policy of never using diathermy at the same time as inflammatory anaesthetic gasses.

Fire
Fire is a rare but nevertheless dangerous hazard. It occurs when pools of spirit used in the preparation of the skin of the patient become ignited. Pools may collect in the umbilicus, axilla or under the patient and it is important that all the spirit should be removed before the diathermy is connected.

Avoidance of hazards
Hazards should be avoided by organising a set routine which is adopted for every patient. Before each operation, the plate and cable should be inspected, and if damaged, discarded. The plate must be carefully applied to the patient at the most suitable site for a particular surgical procedure, hairy areas shaved, and bony areas avoided. The foot piece should be inspected for signs of wear and tear and damage to cables and the patient examined to ensure that no part of the patient's body is in contact with metal objects or equipment. When not in use, during the operation, the live electrode should be kept in a holder made of insulating material.

REFERENCES

D.H.S.S. (1975). Patient safety—surgical diathermy hazards. *Electro-Medical Equipment, Data Sheet*, **EU4**, 1–12.
Dobbie, J. K. (1969). The electrical aspects of surgical diathermy, *Biochemical Engineering*, **4**, 206–216.
Mitchell, J. P. and Lumb, G. N. (1966). *A Handbook of Surgical Diathermy*. John Wright & Sons, Bristol.

7. Irrigating fluids

A. G. England, B.Sc., M.B., Ch.B.

Clear vision is essential to successful transurethral surgery and however good the optical system of the telescope may be, blood will obscure the operating field, unless it is continually washed away.

Typically, each resection will need about five to ten litres of irrigating fluid, although during a long or difficult case, up to twenty litres may be used.

In a busy Urological Centre an average operating list will probably include five or six resections, therefore, large volumes of fluid are required. Tap water has been used for irrigation, but it is now generally accepted that the risk involved in the use of non-sterile fluid is unacceptably high. Intravasation of the irrigating fluid occurs to some extent, during all resections and it has been shown that the volume volume involved can be large (Kumin & Limbert, 1969).

The use of distilled water may result in intravascular haemolysis and renal failure (Creevy, 1947; Drinker et al., 1963; Black), and other complications including dilutional hyponatraemia and cardiac decompensation have also been reported (Ceccarelli & Smitt, 1961; Creevy & Reiser, 1963; Beirne et al., 1965). If the irrigating fluid is not sterile, or contains pyrogenic material, bacteraemia or pyrexia may occur during the post-operative period (Kidd & Burnside, 1965).

It is, therefore, desirable that the irrigating solution should be sterile, pyrogen-free, isotonic, and in order to allow satisfactory diathermy, a non-electrolyte.

Isotonic solutions of dextrose or glycine were found to be rather sticky to use, and experience has shown that haemolysis can be avoided using 2·5 per cent dextrose, 1·1 per cent glycine, or Cytal, a proprietary solution containing 2·7 per cent sorbitol and 0·54 per cent mannitol (Nesbit & Glickman, 1948; Madsen & Madsen, 1965).

Currently, commercial solutions, either in one or three-litre plastic bags, are in general use but the relatively high cost, problems of delivery and storage, as well as the inconvenience associated with the need to replace bags during an operation, has led to considerable interest in alternative methods of supply. In a large hospital, the pharmacy may be able to prepare irrigating solutions more cheaply than commercial preparations, but in general, they are limited to the use of 1 litre glass bottles, which are even less convenient to store and use, than plastic bags.

A number of systems have been designed to supply fluid directly to the operator. These were based on the use of a reservoir tank installed above the theatre, in which a large volume of water was either collected from a still, or sterilised in situ, by means of an electrical heater or high pressure steam. When the water had cooled it was piped to the point of use within the endoscopy theatre.

After the haemolytic complications associated with the use of distilled water became apparent, the systems were modified to include a mixing head which injected a suitable concentrate of dextrose or glycine to produce the irrigating solution. Although convenient for the operator, the difficulty of sterilising the delivery system caused frequent failures (Kelsey & Beeby, 1964).

Bacterial filtration has also been used, but has the disadvantage that the filter may fail silently in use, and no satisfactory method of monitoring the integrity of the membrane has yet been developed (Sykes, 1965). Recently, a new system of water treatment known as reverse-osmosis has been extensively investigated for the treatment of industrial effluents and the production of potable water from brackish or contaminated sources (Leightell, 1971).

The basic process is simple; the water to be treated is forced under high pressure through a semi-permeable membrane (Fig. 7.1). The characteristics of the system depend upon the properties of the membrane, and under controlled conditions, it has been shown that certain commercially available reverse osmosis units consistently

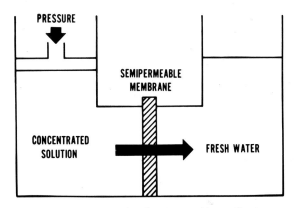

Fig. 7.1 Reverse Osmosis—flow reversed by application of pressure to high concentration solution.

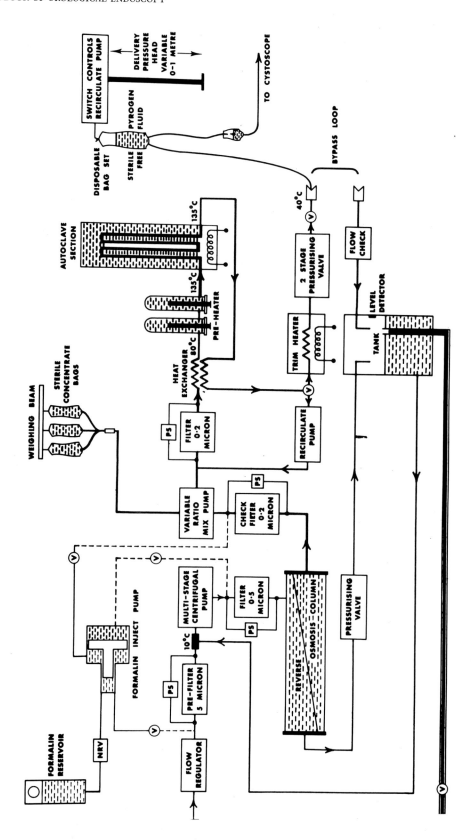

Fig. 7.2   Diagrammatic urological machine.

remove 100 per cent of pyrogenic material and all bacteria from tap water (Palmer & England, 1975). In addition, more than 90 per cent of dissolved solids are removed by the membrane, so that the product water has a relatively high resistivity and is, therefore, satisfactory for diathermy.

The availability of these units has allowed the development of a small machine to produce sterile pyrogen-free solutions for use in the endoscopy theatre.

The system is shown schematically in Figure 7.2. Mains water is passed through the reverse osmosis column by the high pressure pump. The purified water is then mixed with a metered quantity of sterile dextrose or glycine concentrate by a variable ratio proportioning pump. After mixing, the solution passes into a steriliser, in which it is held at a temperature of 135°C for 3 minutes. This ensures sterility, in the event of a failure of the reverse osmosis membrane. A heat exchanger cools the solution to 40°C for delivery to a disposable sterile plastic giving set, hung on an adjustable column, which allows the delivery pressure to be set at the desired level. The machine produces fluid at a maximum rate of 500 mm/minute, which allows the surgeon to work without interruption.

A variety of monitors are included to safeguard the patient against a failure of any critical part of the system, operation is completely automatic, with a programmed flush and pasteurise sequence before operation and a final formalisation phase for storage.

The machine is similar in size to a theatre trolley and allows a pre-packed sterile instrument tray to be placed conveniently for the surgeon's use (Fig. 7.3).

The use of fluid producing machines of this type will not only afford greater convenience to the surgeon, but also, should reduce the incidence of post-operative complications.

Future developments will include modifications to allow the system to be used for continuous flow endoscopy and automatic inflow-outflow monitoring. The process may also be used to produce sterile, pyrogen-free solutions for other medical purposes, for example, bladder irrigation, or at a later date, infusion fluids.

Transurethral surgery requires large volumes of irrigating fluid and this carries significant dangers to the patient unless the operator ensures that this is of the highest quality. The use of non-sterile fluids or of distilled water cannot now be justified.

REFERENCES

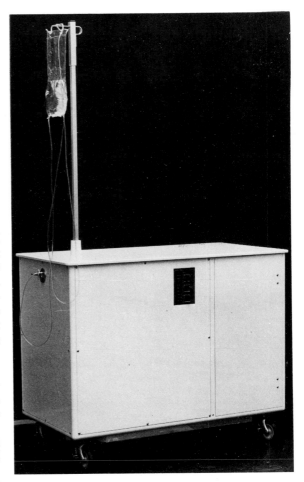

Fig. 7.3   Urological machine—external view.

Beirne, G. J., Madsen, S. O. and Burns, R. O. (1965). Serum electrolyte and osmolarity changes following transurethral resection of the prostate. *Journal of Urology* (Balt.), **93**, 83–86.

Black, D. A. K. Acute renal failure. Chapter 12. *Renal Disease*. Blackwell Scientific Publications, 309–426.

Ceccarelli, F. E. and Smitt, P. C. (1961). Studies on fluid and electrolyte alterations during transurethral prostatectomy. *Journal of Urology* (Balt.), **86**, 434–500.

Creevy, C. D. (1947). Haemolytic reactions during transurethral prostatic resection. *Journal of Urology* (Balt.), **58**, 125–131.

Creevy, C. D. and Reiser, M. P. (1963). The importance of haemolysis in transurethral prostatic resection. Severe and fatal reactions associated with the use of distilled water. *Journal of Urology* (Balt.), **89**, 900–1005.

Drinker, H. R., Shields, T., Grayhoek, S. T. and Laughlin, L. (1963). Simulated transurethral resection reaction in the dog: early signs and optimal treatment. *Journal of Urology* (Balt.), **89**, 595–602.

Kelsey, J. C. and Beeby, M. M. (1964). Sterile water for operating theatres. A trial of tank and piped sterilisers. *Lancet*, **2**, 82.

Kidd, E. E. and Burnside, K. (1965). Bacteraemia, septicaemia and intravascular haemolysis during transurethral resection of the prostate gland. *British Journal of Urology*, **37**, 551–559.

Kunin, S. A. and Limbert, D. J. (1969). Central venous pressure monitoring during transurethral prostatectomy. *Journal of Urology* (Balt.), **102,** 469–472.

Leightell, B. (1971). Horizons widen for reverse osmosis in process engineering. *Process Engineering*, July, 1971.

Madsen, P. O. and Madsen, R. E. (1965). Clinical and experimental evaluation of different irrigating fluids for transurethral surgery. *Investigating Urology*, **3,** 122–129.

Nesbit, R. M. and Glickman, S. T. (1948). The use of glycine as an irrigating solution during transurethral resection. *Journal of Urology* (Balt.), **59,** 1212–1216.

Palmer, C. H. R. and England, A. G. (1975). Problems of pyrogen removal. International Symposium of Pyrogens, *Pharmacology Society*, 1976.

Sykes, G. (1965). *Disinfection and Sterilization*. E. and F. N. Spon Ltd., 2nd edition. London.

8. Normal bladder and urethra

The urinary bladder is a hollow muscular organ with a normal capacity of 250–400 ml of urine situated in the pelvis behind the symphasis pubis. It consists of an outer complicated muscle layer, submucous-alveolar tissue which loosely attaches the muscle layer, which is lined by transitional epithelium, to the underlying mucosa. It is only partially covered by peritoneum on its postero-superior surface. Its blood supply is mainly from the superior and inferior vesical arteries, which form a pre-anastomotic network within its walls especially at the bladder neck.

The two ureters open into the lower part of the bladder at a point which varies between 1–13 cm from the midline. With the internal urethral orifice they form a portion of the bladder known as the trigone, which is bounded by muscular bands each about 4 cm long. The band joining the two ureteric orifices is known as the interureteric bar. The bars joining one ureteric orifice to the other urethral orifice are called the ureteric bars and to the cystoscopist appear to run in the line of the ureter, but, in fact, they are a continuation of the longitudinal muscle fibres of the ureter, Figures 8.1 and 8.2. The shape of the trigone is not constant and often the ureter on one side is displaced, due to the uneven development of the trigone. The mucosa is always smooth and the trigone does not alter, when the bladder is distended, because of its firm fixation to surrounding structures. It is highly vascular, especially at the bladder neck, and care in interpretation must always be exercised so as not to mistake hyperaemia for inflammation.

The air bubble

The air bubble is situated at the highest point of the bladder and is due to air being forced into the bladder during the introduction of the cystoscope. Its size varies with the amount of air introduced and it trembles with every movement of the bladder. It serves as a useful initial landmark for cystoscopists who are in the early stages of training.

Mucous membrane

The normal mucous membrane is pale pink in colour, but it varies from individual to individual, some being pale, others showing a purplish tinge.

The blood vessels

Small vessels, nearly always arteries, can be clearly seen radiating between the mucous membrane and breaking up into delicate tributaries, Figure 8.3. The vascularity of different parts of the bladder varies considerably. The trigone being the most, and the superior part of the fundus the least, vascular. Veins are rarely seen but they can be very prominent.

Bladder musculature

The muscular coat can be seen as discrete strands beneath the mucous membrane, Figure 8.4. Normally, they are few in number, but they can be seen as simple ridges or as patterns, which appear stellate. If the bladder is over distended, the ridges become more prominent and care must be taken to distinguish between this normal trabeculation and that due to bladder neck obstruction.

Ureteric orifices

The ureteric orifices lie at the outer angles of the trigone, where the ureteric and interureteric bars meet. The recognition of the ureteric orifices is the most important part of the bladder examination, as their appearance can give valuable information about kidney pathology which can show itself as excessive activity, inflammation and oedema, ulceration, rigidity and cloudy or haemorrhagic efflux. The typical appearance of a ureteric orifice is that of an ovoid orifice facing upwards and outwards. Frequently blood vessels are seen forming a series of anastomoses in its vicinity. There are, however, many variants from the normal and these can be classified as follows:

Position

Normally the orifice is on the front surface of the bar but it can be on the medial or lateral aspect. It can also be much closer to the bladder neck, a position where it may be difficult to find. The shape depends on the degree of development of the lateral fold and when they are underdeveloped a flat orifice results. If they are overdeveloped the orifice is slit-like and can be difficult to see.

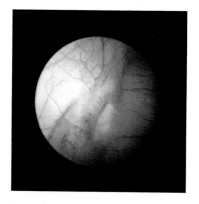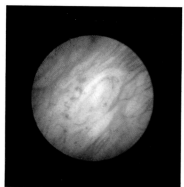

Figs. 8.1 and 8.2
Variants of normal ureteric orifice.

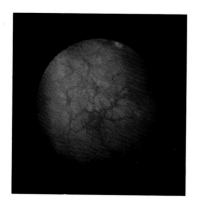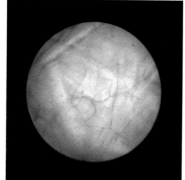

Fig. 8.3
Blood vessels of the bladder.

Fig. 8.4
Bladder muscle.

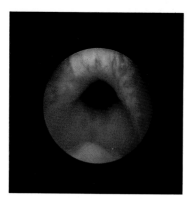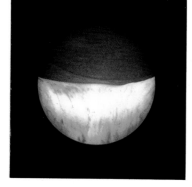

Fig. 8.5
Bladder neck view from the
verumontanum.

Fig. 8.6
Bladder neck at entrance to
the bladder.

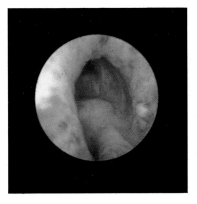

Fig. 8.7
Verumontanum and urethral crest.

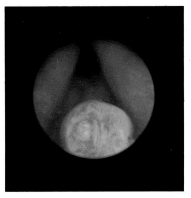

Fig. 8.8
Normal verumontanum.

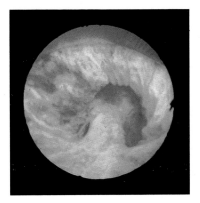

Fig. 8.9
Verumontanum from external
sphincter.

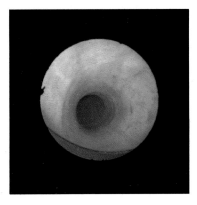

Fig. 8.10
Normal penile urethra.

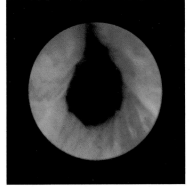

Fig. 8.11
Normal female bladder neck.

Elevation

Infrequently the ureteric orifices appear on the apex of a mound, which can be situated close to the bladder neck, a position where it may be difficult to identify.

Size

The size is variable; some being large, others being small. The small ones may be difficult to identify, unless they are surrounded by blood vessels. When an orifice is about to eject urine, the sides become prominent, the orifice withdraws and then opens as the ureteric peristaltic wave reaches it and the efflux occurs. Indeed, the orifice may be seen first as it opens to eject urine.

THE URETHRA

The male urethra

The male urethra is between 18 and 22 cm long and about 10 mm in diameter. It is divided into 4 separate parts, the prostate, membranous, bulbous and penile.

The prostatic part is 3–4 cm long and runs through the prostate from the bladder neck to the apex. Figures 8.5 and 8.6 show two views of the normal bladder neck, one taken at the level of the verumontanum and the other entering the bladder. On its floor, is a ridge formed by mucous membrane and submucous tissue, called the urethral crest (Fig. 8.7). In the centre of this ridge, the verumontanum forms a prominence on which the orifices of the ejaculatory ducts are situated (Fig. 8.8). It is lined with transitional epithelium as far as

the verumontanum and thereafter by areas of pseudo-stratified columnan and stratified epithelium.

The membranous part of the urethra is the shortest and narrowest part extending from the prostate to the bulb passing through the urogenital diaphragm and being surrounded by the fibres of the external sphincter (Fig. 8.9). It is lined by a combination of pseudo-stratified columns and stratified epithelium.

The bulbous and penile urethra is about 15–16 cm long and extends from the membranous urethra to the external meatus. Except during micturition, the walls are in apposition, apart from the fossa navicularis. It is lined by stratified epithelium except at the tip where the epithelium is stratified squamous in type. Figure 8.10 shows the normal appearance of the penile urethra.

The female urethra

The female urethra is about 5–6 cm long and 6–8 mm in diameter. Except during micturition the anterior and posterior walls of the urethra are in apposition and the mucous membrane appears as a series of longitudinal folds. The centre one on the posterior wall is usually more prominent than the others and is known as the urethral crest. The urethral wall consists of two layers, an outer muscular layer continuous with the bladder and extending the whole length of the tube, and an inner mucous membrane lined by transitional epithelium near the bladder and stratified epithelium close to the vulva. Between the two layers, there is a thin layer of erectile tissue containing a plexus of large veins. Figure 8.11 shows the normal urethra at the bladder neck.

9. Infections of the lower urinary tract

The normal bladder epithelium is remarkably resistant to infection by pyogenic organisms, and therefore, simple, uncomplicated cystitis, is rare. Nevertheless inflammation of the bladder is common, affecting all ages but being more prevalent in the female, during pregnancy or in the presence of some underlying predisposing factor. The most important predisposing factor is a bladder outlet obstruction, which occurs in hypospadias meatal stricture and congenital valves in children and in association with urethral stricture (either post-inflammatory, post-traumatic or neoplastic), meatal stricture, balanitis, prostatic hypertrophy, bladder neck obstruction or prostatic carcinoma in adults. It also occurs as a common complication of spinal cord injury, which is accompanied by retention of urine, due to external sphincter dysfunction. Cystitis may also develop in the presence of a bladder diverticulum, or in females as a complication of cystocoele, a vesical calculus, or foreign bodies introduced per urethra. It almost invariably coexists with malignant bladder tumours, which develop superficial ulceration and necrosis and with vesicocolic fistulae, or following surgical procedures, for example, retained pieces of a catheter or unabsorbed suture material.

A final important factor is direct spread from either the kidney above (pyelitis, pyelonephritis or pyonephrosis), or the urethra below (urethritis, following instrumentation, or coitus).

Infecting organisms

The commonest organism, accounting for about 90% of infection is the Escherichia coli. Other organisms such as Proteus Vulgaria, Pseudomonas Pyocyaneus, Streptococcus Faecalis and Staphylococcus Aureus and Albus may also be found and rarely, Klebsiella and Candida Albicans.

Investigation

It is essential that a definitive diagnosis is made before specific treatment is started and this is especially important in the mild type of case as there are many conditions which simulate the symptoms of cystitis:

1. Conditions giving rise to excessive quantities of urine such as glycosuria and chronic nephritis
2. Diseases of neighbouring organs such as urethritis

and prostatis in the male and cervicitis and parametritis in the female; also enlargement of the uterus and ovarian cysts pressing on the bladder can give rise to pain and frequency.

This aspect should be kept constantly in mind, in the investigation of cases of lower urinary tract infection, and the presence or absence of pus in a midstream specimen of urine is important evidence. It was a salutary experience to find, during an investigation carried out with the co-operation of a group of general practitioners that 50 per cent of patients presented with symptoms of 'cystitis' had a sterile urine, with less than 10 leucocytes per high power field in the first specimen of urine examined. In addition to the urine analysis, a full investigation must be carried out so that underlying predisposing factors can be diagnosed and either corrected or eliminated. One of the important investigations is a cystoscopy, but it must be stressed immediately, that it is unwise and may even be dangerous to carry out this examination in the presence of an acute infection. The bladder appearance will be studied under the following headings:

1. Changes in the mucous membrane.
2. Vascular changes.

Changes in the mucous membrane

In the acute phase, the mucous membrane, normally a pale pink colour becomes intensely hyperanaemic and bright red. This may involve either the whole or only part of the bladder wall. Figure 9.1 shows an acute patchy cystitis. When the inflammation has become chronic, the mucosa become elevated, almost polypoidal and appear as exuberant granulation tissue. These lesions are best seen around fistulae or malignant tumours (Fig. 9.2), and are sometimes very difficult to distinguish from acute tuberculous lesions, so that a biopsy will always be required.

Oedema invariably occurs in cystitis, but it is not so noticeable in the early stages. It is usually manifested by small bullae, smooth, round, dome-shaped, with translucent walls, containing a watery exudate. They may, rarely, be simple, but it is more usual to find them as a conglomerate mass, like a bunch of grapes (Fig. 9.3). They can be situated anywhere but are usually found on the base of the bladder or close to a ureteric

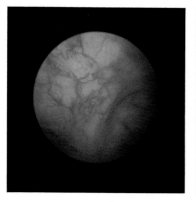

Fig. 9.1
Simple patchy cystitis.

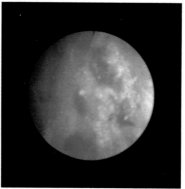

Fig. 9.2
Inflammation surrounding a carcinoma of the bladder.

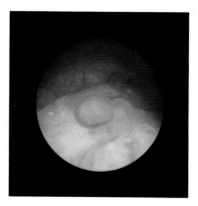

Fig. 9.3
Cystitis cystica.

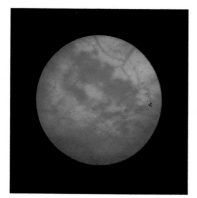

Fig. 9.4
Haemorrhagic cystitis.

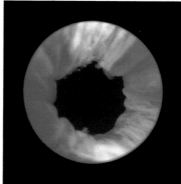

Fig. 9.5
Polypi at the bladder neck in the female.

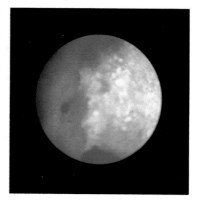

Fig. 9.6
Cystitis with fibrophosphatic deposits.

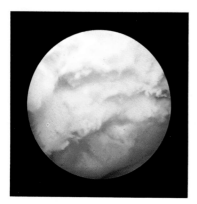

Fig. 9.7
Encrusted cystitis.

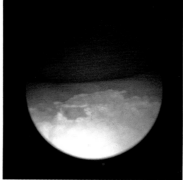

Fig. 9.8
Leucoplakia on the base of the bladder.

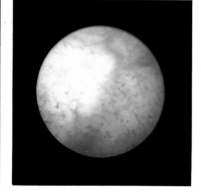

Fig. 9.9
Irradiation cystitis.

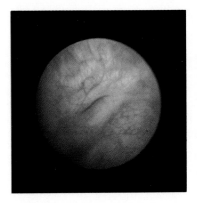

Fig. 9.10
Early tuberculosis of a ureteric
orifice.

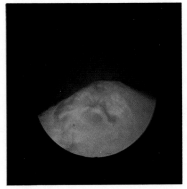

Fig. 9.11
Granulations around a ureteric
orifice.

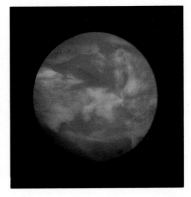

Fig. 9.12
Tuberculous ulcer.

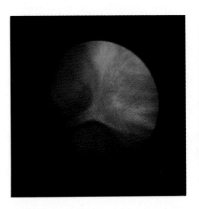

Fig. 9.13
Healed tuberculous cystitis

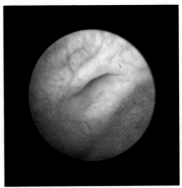

Fig. 9.14
Healing tuberculous ureteric
orifice.

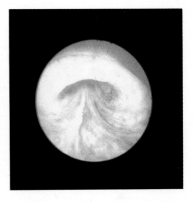

Fig. 9.15
Healing tuberculous ureteric
orifice.

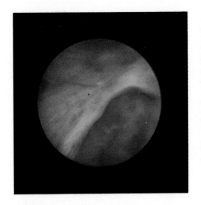

Fig. 9.16
Healing tuberculous cystitis with
scarring.

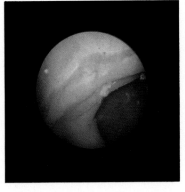

Fig. 9.17
Caecocystoplasty showing demarcation
between bladder and caecum.

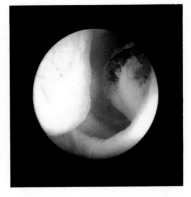

Fig. 9.18
Tuberculous prostatic cavity containing
calculi.

orifice and they most commonly occur in chronic Escherichia Coli infection.

Vascular changes

Vascular changes are the earliest manifestation of cystitis. In the very early stages, the vessels enlarge and become more obvious, produce an area bright red in colour. This may be simple, multiple, or involve most of the mucous membrane. As the dilatation progresses the vessels further increase in size, rupture and produce small punctate haemorrhages (Fig. 9.4). In later stages, it is impossible to distinguish individual vessels, and the area of the bladder wall infected, appears completely covered by vascular tissue.

Treatment

In the treatment of an acute urinary tract infection, the first essential is, to isolate the organism and discover its antibiotic sensitivity spectrum, and so, a clean mid-stream specimen of urine must be sent to the laboratory for analysis. It is desirable to await the result of the urine culture before starting antibiotic treatment, but often this is not possible, as the patient's symptoms, when first seen, are too severe. It is, therefore, important to know, which antibiotics are most likely to be effective and repeated surveys of all first specimens of urine submitted for analysis to laboratories have shown that, of the oral antibiotics 98 per cent of organisms were sensitive to Trimethoprim (Septrin, Bactrim), 95 per cent to Nalidixic acid (Negram), 90 per cent to Nitro-furantoin (Furadantin) and only 60 per cent to Ampicillin (Penbritin). If the infection is severe enough to warrant parenteral treatment the antibiotic of choice is Genta-mycin as the same survey showed that 100 per cent of organisms were sensitive to this antibiotic. It is import-ant, not only to give adequate doses but to continue the treatment for ten to fourteen days. In all cases, a high fluid intake should be encouraged, as a high urinary output decreases the concentration of organisms. Once the acute phase is passed, a full investigation of the urinary tract must be carried out and any underlying abnormalities treated. If it is the first attack of infection, urinanalysis should be carried out two to three months after the treatment has finished. If the urine has remained sterile, the patient can be discharged. If, however, it still remains infected, further supervision must be con-tinued. Even after the satisfactory treatment of under-lying abnormalities, there remain a few cases, in whom the infection frequently recurs, and in these, long-term chemotherapy may be necessary. Low dose chemo-therapy taken last thing at night and continued for six months or longer has given excellent results in many patients.

Other forms of cystitis

Urethrotrigonitis

This is a condition which is very common in females, occurring usually after the menopause; one which is easy to treat but very difficult to cure. Most patients present with increased frequency of micturition, nocturia and occasional initial haematuria. The cause is unknown, but it has been suggested that it is due to obstruction in the submucous glands around the bladder neck. On urethroscopy, polypi are seen surrounding the internal meatus (Fig. 9.5), and there may also be an inflamed and oedematous mucous membrane spreading on to the base of the bladder. In some cases, a narrowing of the external urinary meatus is present and there may even be a bladder neck obstruction. Periodic urethral dilata-tion at three to six monthly intervals may help some of the patients and others are improved by diathermy fulguration of the bladder neck polypi. This surgical management can be combined with an oral oestrogen such as Pentovis 0·25 mg t.d.s. for four weeks, repeated, after an interval, if necessary, especially if there is evidence of coincidental atrophy of the vaginal mucous membrane.

Encrusted cystitis

This is a rare form of cystitis due to the chronic infection with Bacillus Proteus, which can be most intractable. The bladder becomes contracted, the mucous membrane is oedematous and is covered by plaques of phosphatic material (Figs. 9.6 and 9.7). The encrustations are difficult to dislodge, but when they are detached, severe bleeding can occur. The urine is invariably alkaline and contains blood, phosphatic debris, mucous and numerous leucocytes. The condi-tion may be accompanied by bladder neck obstruction, which must be corrected. Treatment consists of acetic acid bladder irrigation, acidification of the urine with either ammonium chloride or ascrobic acid, 1 gm of each being given once or twice a day, and prolonged chemotherapy with an appropriate drug, Negram being the first choice.

Leucoplakia

The normal epithelium in the bladder is transitional, as, although stratified, it never becomes keratinised under normal conditions. However, under certain circum-stances, the cells undergo metaplasia and the result is leucoplakia. It is a rare condition, and is invariably accompanied by signs of chronic cystitis and should be regarded as a hyperplastic response of the tissues to long-standing infection. The urine may or may not contain organisms but invariably there are a large number of leucocytes in each specimen, together with quantities of stratified epithelium. Urine examination is, therefore, likely to be very helpful and may even diagnose the condition before cystoscopy. It must be considered a precancerous condition.

The patch is usually seen at the bladder neck, is silvery in colour, smooth, variable in size, with an irregular outline, sharply defined edges and no granulations or fissures (Fig. 9.8). In view of the risk of malignant change the whole area should be removed, endoscopic diathermy excision being the method of choice.

Irradiation cystitis

Symptoms of cystitis are nearly always experienced after irradiation of the bladder. In most cases they disappear spontaneously, but occasionally, they persist and become severe and intractable. In particular, severe haematuria occurs, which poses many problems. The bladder becomes contracted and the cystoscopic appearance shows haemorrhagic areas scattered over a pale atrophic mucous membrane (Fig. 9.9). Local treatment was invariably unsuccessful, but recently, satisfactory treatment has been reported using Helmstein's technique.

GENITOURINARY TUBERCULOSIS

Although the incidence of genitourinary tuberculosis has been steadily declining during the last decade, epidemics of new cases are still being reported. These continue to pose problems, especially if treatment is unsatisfactory; a state, which applies particularly to under-developed areas, where the control of chemotherapy is difficult and often inadequate.

Tuberculosis of the kidney is always caused by a metabolic spread of organisms via the blood stream; the primary focus, in nearly every case, being in the chest. These organisms produce small foci in close proximity to the glomeruli. Some heal, but the majority expand, ulcerate into part of the collecting system, producing a tuberculous bacilluria. These lesions can go on increasing in size, causing the classical ulcer-cavernous lesion, and may spread even further producing a complete destruction of renal parenchyma. Organisms pass down the ureter and into the bladder, causing lesions which are always secondary to renal tuberculosis. In the bladder, the infection starts around one or other ureteric orifice, which initially may appear as a red inflamed area (Fig. 9.10). Later, the inflammation becomes more acute and bullous granulations develop, which may obscure the ureteric orifice (Fig. 9.11). These granulations may spread on to the base of the bladder or to the lateral wall. From these lesions, organisms can spread and cause typical tuberculous cystitis in any part of the bladder. If the disease

progresses further granulations may proceed to a shallow ulcer with irregular edges and a yellow slough in the base (Fig. 9.12). Ultimately, these ulcers involve the muscle, which becomes replaced by fibrous tissue, producing a stellate appearance due to fibrous contractions (Fig. 9.13). Small areas of inflammation appear on the surface of these fibrous bands until healing is complete. Tubercles may be seen, but if so, they are close to the ureteric orifice. They are, however, excessively rare, and have only been seen by the author on two occasions.

Treatment

There have been many outstanding milestones in the treatment of tuberculosis, amongst those can be included the discovery of streptomycin and isoniazid, and the appreciation that combinations of drugs prevent the emergence of resistant strains, and that short course chemotherapy can be considered a satisfactory method of treatment. For the last eighteen months, the standard régime of treatment for genitourinary tuberculosis has been a course of rifampicin 450 mg, isoniazid 300 mg and pyrozinamide 1 gm given daily for two to three months. At the end of this period, the treatment was continued with pyrozinamide $1\frac{1}{2}$ gm rifampicin 900 mg, taken twice a week in two equally divided doses for three or four months. This treatment has been extremely effective and no reversions have been experienced up to the first six months after completion of the treatment. If there is a serious bladder lesion, this treatment can cause rapid improvement, so that a ureteric orifice previously invisible, because of granulations, can be seen as an inflamed oedematous orifice. As healing further progresses, the ureteric orifice becomes involved in fibrous tissue and appears withdrawn and rigid (Figs. 9.14 and 9.15). Such a ureter can either produce reflux or obstruction, and if the fibrosis continues, becomes classically known as the golf hole ureter, something which is now, rarely, seen. If the inflammation has been very severe before treatment is commenced, the bladder can heal; but the bladder is always distorted by bands of fibrous tissue (Fig. 9.16), and the whole of the bladder covered by tuberculous granulations, healing is much slower and there is always contraction of the bladder due to intramuscular fibrosis with a capacity reduced to 50 to 100 ml. In these cases, bladder enlargement has to be carried out. Caecocystoplasty is favoured by the author for this procedure and Figure 9.17 shows the results of such a procedure, revealing the difference between the normal bladder and the attached caecum. At the end of the latter period of time the velvety appearance of the caecum adopts a smoother appearance, much more like a bladder mucous membrane, and occasionally, it is very difficult to tell the difference between the two types of epithelium. Occasionally, the disease involves the prostate and if the destruction of the tissue is extensive a cavity, in which calculi develop, results. Figure 9.18 shows a cavity containing calculi. The only satisfactory treatment is to perform an endoscopic prostatic resection, and remove the calculi with foreign body forceps.

REFERENCES

Helmstein, K. (1972). Treatment of bladder carcinoma by hydrostatic pressure technique. Report on 43 cases. *British Journal of Urology*, **44,** 434.

Kunin, C. M. (1974). *Detection, Prevention and Management of Urinary Tract Infection*. Second Edition, Lea & Febiger, Philadelphia.

10. The prostate and urethra

THE PROSTATE

The prostate gland is the romantic organ in urology, as throughout the centuries the treatment of the pathological changes has produced ideas of vision and inspiration, yet, despite all the advances, it still provides a fertile field for research.

Benign prostatic hypertrophy

Benign prostatic hypertrophy usually occurs in the male after the 5th decade of life, and only a small percentage present with symptoms earlier. The effects produced are due to bladder outlet obstruction, and are known, collectively, as prostatism. The most important symptom is difficulty in starting micturition coupled with a diminishing stream. In addition, the patient complains of increasing frequency of micturition, especially at night, occasional dysuria and haematuria. Gradually the condition deteriorates; a feeling of urgency is not uncommon and initial and terminal dribbling may occur. In a few cases, the patient presents with an acute urinary retention.

As the prostate enlarges, the posterior urethra becomes elongated and diminished in diameter and the appearances vary according to size of the prostate. Figure 10.1 shows an early enlargement of lateral lobes of the prostate, which is confined almost entirely to the posterior urethra. In these cases, the anterior angle is often quite wide and the middle lobe is only marginally hypertrophied. As the enlargement increases, all the tissue in the lateral lobes becomes involved and the anterior angle is narrow, invariably less than 90°. In this type of prostatic hypertrophy, the middle lobe is often partially hidden by the lateral lobes, but it must always be identified before a prostatic resection is commenced. To do this, it may be necessary, to increase the pressure of the irrigating fluid. As the instrument passes through the lateral lobes, the floor of the urethra appears to lift until the middle lobe comes into view. In some cases, the lateral lobes are small, but the middle lobe is so hypertrophied that it occludes the field and acts as a ball valve. In other cases, the lateral lobes are slightly enlarged and blend into the middle lobe, which then obscures the view into the bladder (Figs. 10.2 & 10.3). The endoscope passes over the middle lobe which slopes abruptly down to the base of the bladder. If, however, the lobe is large, it may be impossible to see either the ureteric orifice, or the prostatic recess. When the bladder neck obstruction is severe, typical bladder changes will be revealed as well as the classical appearances of a compensatory hypertrophy of the bladder muscle. Trabeculation, both fine and coarse, and also pseudo-diverticulae and cellules will be seen (Figs. 10.4 & 10.5). Occasionally, by looking carefully into the prostatic recess, calculi may be observed.

The treatment is prostatectomy, preferably by transurethral resection. Figure 10.6 shows a healed cavity after such a procedure, with the typical honeycomb appearance of the capsule.

Prostatic carcinoma

Carcinoma of the prostate is discovered in approximately 20 per cent of males over the age of 60. It may be found in an apparently normal gland or in one which has begun to hypertrophy. The disease often remains dormant for a long time and produces no symptoms, but, frequently, is only found, when the pathologist examines sections from an excised gland.

The prostatic carcinoma may also arise as a nodule in the periphery of the gland, close to the capsule, and becomes an advanced growth by the time it reaches the prostatic urethra. When the growth commences in the lateral lobes, it usually invades the urethra earlier and gives rise to symptoms of prostatism. When it advances further, pain may be felt in the pelvic areas and lumbar regions. On cystoscopy, particularly in the early stages, it is difficult to identify the lesion. The tissue appears whiter (Fig. 10.7), and is different from the normal 'cheesy' appearance of resected prostatic tissue. A fibrous prostate appears similar, and the pathologist is then left to make the definitive diagnosis. As the lesion advances the prostatic urethra becomes rigid and the disease ulcerates through the mucous membrane, appearing as an irregular surface with haemorrhagic areas. As the disease progresses, undermining the base of the bladder, and areas become irregular, there may be superficial ulceration. In all cases, the normal architecture of the prostate disappears and is replaced by amorphous haemorrhagic tissue.

When the bladder is invaded and appears inflamed, it may be difficult to tell whether the bladder or

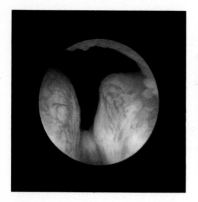

Fig. 10.1
Prostatic hypertrophy, lateral lobe.

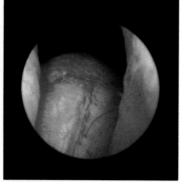

Fig. 10.2
Prostatic hypertrophy, middle lobe.

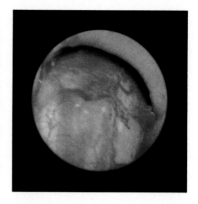

Fig. 10.3
Prostatic hypertrophy, middle lobe.

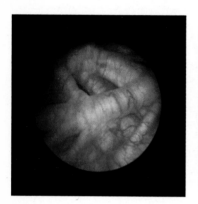

Fig. 10.4
Gross bladder trabeculation.

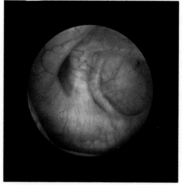

Fig. 10.5
Gross bladder trabeculation with pseudodiverticulum.

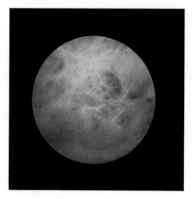

Fig. 10.6
Healed cavity after transurethral resection of prostate.

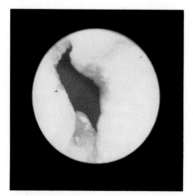

Fig. 10.7
Carcinoma of the prostate.

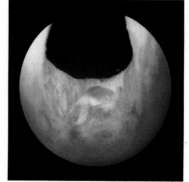

Fig. 10.8
Bladder neck sclerosis.

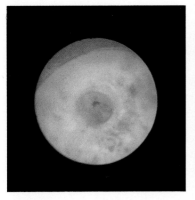

Fig.10.9
Urethral stricture, small lumen.

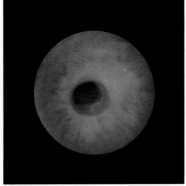

Fig. 10.10
Urethral stricture, short
annular.

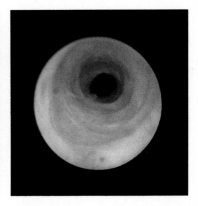

Fig. 10.11
Urethral stricture, long annular.

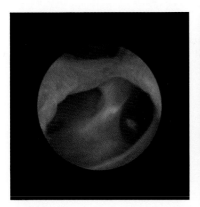

Fig. 10.12
False passages in the posterior
urethra.

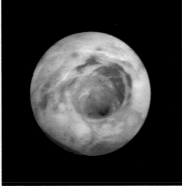

Fig. 10.13
Appearance of urethral stricture after
dilatation.

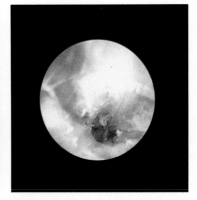

Fig. 10.14
Carcinoma of the urethra.

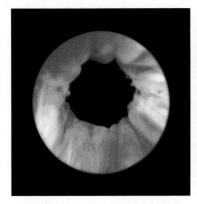

Fig. 10.15
Bladder neck polyps at the lateral
urethral orifice in the female.

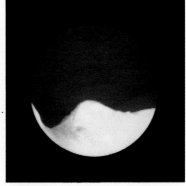

Fig. 10.16
Malignant tumour at the bladder
neck in the female.

prostate is the primary lesion. In these cases, a biopsy is mandatory, in order to determine the best line of treatment.

Bladder neck contracture

Mitchell 1955 describes two types of bladder neck obstruction. In the first there is a large subcervical pouch with a fibrous base rising at the bladder neck with minimal enlargement of the lateral lobes. On cystoscopy, this lesion appears as a tight ring (Fig. 10.8). The second type is due to a thickened bladder neck, which can be readily felt, on rectal examination, against the examining cystoscope. The thickening may involve the lateral lobes of the prostate, giving the impression of a narrowing of the urethra. In both of these conditions, resection of prostatic tissue is rarely necessary, and satisfactory relief of symptoms can be achieved by lateral incision, with a diathermy probe, at three and nine o'clock positions, of the bladder neck. As the incision deepens, the bladder neck gapes widely. It is important that the incisions are continued right through the sclerotic tissue.

THE URETHRA

Ever since enquiring minds have probed into the functions of the human body, the urethra has been constantly discussed. Even Aristotle and Hippocrates talked about problems of infections and bougies were mentioned in historical studies of Ancient Egypt. It is understandable therefore that lesions of the urethra assume a place of high importance in urological problems and demand a high degree of gentleness and skill, for nowhere is Moynihan's adage 'that tissues should be caressed' more applicable.

Urethral pathology—male

Congenital abnormalities

Congenital diverticulae may be found in the adult male, but are much more commonly seen in the child. In the adult, the diagnosis may be suspected, if the patients complain of dribbling after micturition, which is caused by the diverticulum emptying into the urethra immediately after the main urinary stream has ceased. These diverticulae are nearly always in the anterior urethra and the opening may be large or small. The large opening is readily seen on urethroscopy, but the narrow neck variety is easily missed and is better demonstrated by urethrography.

Inflammation

As organisms are invariably to be found in the urethra it is surprising that urethritis does not occur more frequently. However, most of these organisms are non-pathogenic and when an infection occurs it is due to specific organisms, the commonest of which is the Gonococcus. Gonococcal urethritis rapidly responds to treatment and a very effective method is the single intramuscular injection of 2·4 megaunits of Procaine Penicillin. A Trichomonas infection should not be forgotten, as the symptoms are soon controlled with a seven day course of metronidazole 200 mgm, 8 hourly for 7–10 days. Non-specific urethritis is now being seen more frequently and is easy to treat, but difficult to cure. A combination of Tetracycline and Erythromycin 250 mgm each q.d.s. for 14 days is the best treatment, but if unsuccessful, can be changed to Erythromycin 250 mgm q.d.s. given with Spiramycin 500 mgm q.d.s. for 7–10 days. Sometimes, if these two fail, a combination of Tetracycline 500 mgm q.d.s. and Streptomycin 1 gm daily given for 14 days is successful.

Urethral stricture

Most strictures of the urethra are either inflammatory or traumatic.

Inflammatory strictures

The majority of inflammatory strictures occur as a late sequel to gonococcal infection, which is becoming less common since the introduction of adequate chemotherapy, and the abandoning of the instillation into the urethra of local irritant antiseptics, as a method of treatment. These strictures nearly always occur in the anterior urethra and may be rubbery or densely fibrotic, depending on the intensity of the infection. They are caused by the replacement of the mucosa and submucous layers and eventually the muscle coat by fibrous tissue. This leads to narrowing of the urethra, with almost complete obstruction of the lumen. Tuberculosis is also a rare cause of urethral stricture in the membranous urethra. This is hardly ever seen now that chemotherapeutic treatment of the primary lesion is so satisfactory. Inflammatory strictures may have a small lumen (Fig. 10.9), be short and annular (Fig. 10.10) or involve the ureter for more than 5 cm (Fig. 10.11).

Traumatic strictures

Traumatic strictures are now more common than those due to infection and there are three main causes.

Perineal injury

The classical cause of this type of injury is when a man falls astride a sharp edge such as the traditional up-turned manhole cover. This produces a short stricture in the first part of the bulbous urethra and is accompanied by bruising the haemorrhage in the perineum.

Fractured pelvis

A severe fracture of the pelvis results in disrupion of the membranous urethra, which in many cases results in separation of the two ends by quite a large margin, the prostate being forced into the pelvis with the bladder. Failure to carry out satisfactory treatment, as soon as possible after the initial injury, is the main cause of the difficult late stricture.

Instrumental

Misfortune during an endoscopic procedure is a rare cause of stricture. It is much more likely, if an in-dwelling cathether is used without due cause, and especially if it is kept in place by elastoplasty which is wound too tightly round the penis. In this way, pressure of the catheter against the urethra can result in avascular necrosis of the urethral mucosa, which heals by fibrosis and stricture.

Management

Once it has been accepted that urethroscopy is the initial part of an endoscopic examination, false passages due to blind bouginage (Fig. 10.12), should never occur, and blind bouginage as an initial procedure is to be condemned, especially as modern sophisticated urological instruments are now available. The urethroscopy should reveal the stricture at the first examination and it is often possible to direct the small panendoscope through the stricture. Should this manoeuvre fail, a filiform bougie passed down the urethroscope can often be manipulated through the stricture under direct vision. The urethroscope is then withdrawn and the stricture is dilated by screwing on to the first filiform, bougies of gradually increasing size. Once the filiform bougie has been passed through the stricture, an alternative method of treatment is to carry out an internal urethrotomy under direct vision, using either a diathermy or short urethrotomy knife. The incisions are made at the 12 o'clock position, incising the fibrous tissue until the urethra ceases to gape and long or short strictures can be treated equally well. Once the stricture has been adequately dilated, the examination of the urethra is completed, and the stricture, which can be either long or short, assessed. Even though urethroplasty has reached such a high degree of excellence, gentle and careful bouginage still remains the best treatment for many strictures. Even so, there is inevitable trauma (Fig. 10.13), and it is small wonder that strictures recur.

Urethral tumours

Malignant urethral tumours are rare and are usually found in the proximal urethra (Fig. 10.14); the majority are squamous cell carcinoma and the prognosis is poor, less than 15 per cent surviving 5 years. Radical cysto-urethrectomy with urinary diversion offers the best chance of survival.

Urethral pathology—female

The urethral syndrome

Many female patients present with recurring symptoms of frequency and dysuria, for which no cause can be found. Such a complex has been misguidedly called the urethral syndrome, as there is no conclusive evidence that the urethra is the cause. Organisms are rarely isolated from the urine yet on urethroscopy the urethra is inflamed and there are often numerous polyps surrounding the bladder neck (Fig. 10.15). Many patients are relieved by repeated urethral dilatation with or without urethrotomy of the bladder neck, performed at the 3 and 9 o'clock positions, with the Otis urethrotome. Others are temporarily improved by small doses of oestrogen, especially if there is evidence of coincidental senile vagination. Although helpful, both of these methods are empirical and the cause of the problem still remains unsolved.

Malignant tumours

The incidence of malignant tumours is comparable to that of the male and the majority are squamous carcinoma. They progress slowly and many have spread outside the urethra before the patients present for treatment. In the early stages, frequency, dysuria and urgency are the common symptoms, but if the lesion is more extensive, haematuria is the main feature. It is essential that a biopsy should be taken of all tumours and Figure 10.16 shows an early squamous carcinoma at the bladder neck. In early tumours, the treatment of choice is interstitial irradiation with gold seeds and there is a 40 per cent, 5 year cure. For more advanced cases, cystourethrectomy with urinary diversion is suggested as the best line of treatment, but the outlook is very poor, less than 10 per cent of patients surviving for five years.

11. Unusual bladder pathology

CHRONIC INTERSTITIAL CYSTITIS (HUNNERS ULCER)

Chronic interstitial cystitis is a disease which predominantly affects females over the age of forty. The cause is unknown, but it is thought to be due to an autoimmune reaction, as antibodies to the human bladder have been found in some patients.

Symptoms
Many patients present with intense intractable lower abdominal and perineal pain, often worse on sitting; day and night frequency of micturition and dysuria are common, and in severe cases, haematuria is always found. These symptoms can be caused by any severe cystitis, but the difference between the two, is the severity of the symptoms produced by relatively small bladder lesions.

Cystoscopic appearance
The bladder capacity is invariably reduced in the early stages. One or two inflamed areas, with a central yellow slough, which ultimately becomes a scar, are seen, usually on the base of the bladder, but as the condition progresses, the bladder becomes fibrosed and forms a stellate appearance, on the surface of which, the epithelium is oedematous and inflamed. These changes have spread to the fundus of the bladder and Figures 11.1 and 11.2 show two such areas, which tend to bleed on overdistension.

Differential diagnosis
In the early stages the lesion can be confused with carcinoma *in situ*, but as the disease progresses tuberculosis and Bilharzia must be excluded. In all cases a biopsy should be taken, but if the changes are seen in the fundus, and if the ureteric orifices are normal, tuberculosis can be excluded, as tuberculosis of the bladder is always secondary to a focus in the kidney.

Treatment
The results of treatment are far from satisfactory, and the many methods that have been tried only emphasise that there is no generally accepted standard treatment. Bladder distension, has given the best results in the author's hands. The technique adopted is to distend the bladder by a special balloon, up to a pressure of the patient's diastolic pressure + 10 mm mercury. Under continuous epidural anaesthesia, the pressure is continued for half an hour and then released. This procedure is repeated four times at each session. This technique has the merit of being relatively simple and can be repeated again and again if the symptoms recur. Bladder transection and enterocystoplasty have been reported to give good results in some cases, but these are formidable surgical procedures, and should only be considered when the simpler measures have failed.

BLADDER DIVERTICULAE

The large majority of bladder diverticulae are secondary to urinary outflow obstruction and occur in males over the age of 50. They are situated on the base of the bladder, close to one or other ureteric orifice, and they may be multiple or single. They can distend to a large size, even equalling the capacity of the bladder itself. When they are small, they must be distinguished from the shallow cellules, which are seen between the trabeculae of the hypertrophied bladder. The wall consists largely of mucous membrane covered by fibrous tissue. There is almost a complete absence of muscle in the wall, so that it cannot contract and empty the contents. The cystoscopic appearance is that of a punched hole in the bladder wall, which appears small and irregular, when the bladder is emptied, but which becomes smoother and wider, as the bladder fills, with a rolled edge due to the muscular ring (Fig. 11.2).

Symptoms
Diverticulae do not give rise to symptoms *per se*. The patient's symptoms are due either to bladder outlet obstruction, lower urinary tract infection or a combination of both, and the diagnosis is made by radiology and confirmed by cystoscopy.

Treatment
The treatment is diverticulectomy, which is nearly always performed at the same time as the surgical treatment of bladder outlet obstruction. It can be carried out by extra or infravesical dissection, or by

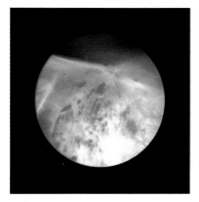

Fig. 11.1
Hunners ulcer.

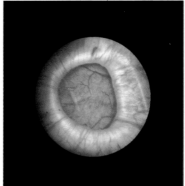

Fig. 11.2
Diverticulum.

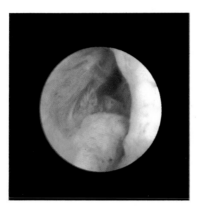

Fig. 11.3
Tumour arising in diverticulum.

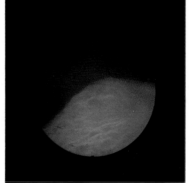

Fig. 11.4
Inflamed oedematous ureteric
orifice.

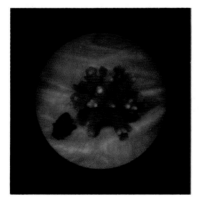

Fig. 11.5
Bizarre bladder calculus.

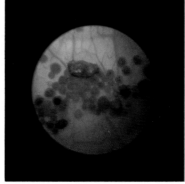

Fig. 11.6
Multiple small bladder calculi.

intravesical invagination, depending on the presence or absence of infection.

Complications

There are 3 common complications; infection, calculus formation and malignant change. Infection and calculi are easily diagnosed but neoplasms may be difficult to see, and it is, therefore, important to introduce the cystoscope into the diverticulum and carry out a thorough examination at the time of the initial cystoscopy. Figure 11.3 shows an early carcinoma, arising in the wall of a diverticulum.

VESICAL CALCULI

Vesical calculi are either primary or secondary. The primary calculi have become rare, whereas the secondary, are now commonly seen.

Most secondary calculi arise in the kidney, and provided that there is no outflow obstruction are voided spontaneously in the urine, especially in the female. Occasionally, they become lodged in the interminal part of the ureter close to the bladder neck, producing inflammation and oedema (Fig. 11.4). The commonest predisposing factors in the male are prostatic enlargement, bladder neck obstruction, recurrent attacks of severe cystitis, carcinoma, diverticulae, urethral stricture and the neurogenic disturbances of bladder function. In the female, they occur secondary to bladder neck obstruction, carcinoma, or a cystocoele. In both sexes, they form over foreign bodies, such as retained suture material or the balloon of an indwelling catheter.

Composition

Most calculi are made up of a mixture of calcium phosphate, magnesium and oxalate in varying quantities, depending on the pH of the urine. Pure uric acid stones are rare and are completely translucent to X-ray. Cystine and other metabolic stones are also rare, and are soft and only give a faint shadow on X-ray.

Symptoms

Calculi may be symptomless, and only be discovered accidentally. The classical symptom is pain felt at the tip of the penis, which is aggravated by movement and relieved by lying down. These symptoms are now rarely encountered, and the patients, in whom calculi are found, are usually being investigated for a mild or severe urinary tract infection. Rarely, they may present with retention of urine due to the calculus becoming impacted in the urethra.

Size

The size and shape of calculi are very variable. The assessment of the size is important, as on an accurate determination, depends the decision, as to the best method of treatment. Radiographic estimation may be misleading, unless it is remembered that the size on the X-ray film is 10–12 per cent larger than the actual size.

Management

The management will be dictated by the result of the investigations carried out, but in every case, the patient should have all the routine investigations, which are mandatory for patients presenting with calculi anywhere in the urinary tract.

In considering treatment there are two aspects. First, to deal with any predisposing factors, such as bladder neck obstruction, or urethral stricture, and secondly to remove the calculi. There are few calculi, which cannot be destroyed by the lithotrite, and the fragments evacuated, but there are occasional cases, in which the calculus is so big, that a cystolithotomy has to be performed. In those cases, where the patient presents with an oedematous ureteric orifice, careful resection of the oedematous tissue with a resectoscope may reveal the calculus, which can then be removed without difficulty.

Bizarre shaped calculi and multiple small stones are seen in patients with prostatic hypertrophy (Figs. 11.5 & 11.6).

BILHARZIA

Bilharzia has been a scourge of Egypt for thousands of years, ova having been found by Ruffer in the urinary tract of mummies dating back to the XXth Dynasty 1200–1085 BC. About 60 per cent of the 40 million people who populate Egypt have been infected, at one time or another, and the complications that occur, often pose insuperable problems, for the urologist. It is, predominantly, a male disease, so much so that because of the frequent haematuria the Egyptians have been called 'the race of menstruating males'. The discovery of the worm was made by Theodore Bilharz in 1851, when he was carrying out a postmortem examination on an Egyptian boy. It was, however, many years later that Leiper identified the snail, which was essential, as an intermediate host, to complete the life cycle of the worm.

Cycle of bilharzia

The worm that is responsible for Bilharzia of the urinary tract is the Schistosoma Haematobium, a Trematode measuring 10–11 mm in length and 2 mm in breadth. So as to be able to enter small venules, the body of the male enfolds itself like a canoe to form the gynaecophoric canal, in which lodges, the longer, but much thinner, female. Both the male and female worms form in the liver from the cercariae, and enter the portal venous system, where they continue to mature. They swim against the stream, enter the superior and inferior mesenteric veins and ultimately reach the vesical veins through the superior rectal veins. Mating of the male and female worm takes place in the more peripheral veins. At this stage, the female leaves the male and being thinner makes its way into the smaller venules, which abound in the bladder submucosa, and there lays her eggs. The eggs pass through the mucous membrane, into the bladder, by the combined effect of proleolytic enzymes excreted by the egg and the contractions of the bladder muscle, and are then voided in the urine, as it is essential for the completion of the cycle that the ova leave the human body. This part of the cycle takes 10–12 weeks from the time of infection. Once the ova reach the water, the miracidia contained in the egg hatch, and immediately search for their host, the snail Bullinus Truncatus. The miracidia do not live more than 48 hours, so, it is essential, that they find their host within this period, or the cycle will be broken. The miracidia attack the snail, penetrate and make their way to the liver, where they develop into cercariae. All this takes about 6 weeks. As the cercariae develop, cystic spaces form, ultimately burst, and discharge large numbers of cercariae into the water. The cercariae measure about 6 mm in length and consist of a head, a forked tail, with which they swim, seeking their definitive host, usually man. The life span of the cercariae is also short, less than 48 hours, so that a host must be found within this period, if the cycle is to be completed. Once they find their host, they pierce the skin, shed their tails, enter the systemic circulation and are then disseminated to all parts of the body. Only those, which enter the portal system, survive, and produce the adult worms, which then migrate to initiate the sexual phase of the life cycle. Very little is known about the activities of the adult worms once they have mated and produced their eggs. It is likely that, the female after laying her eggs makes her way back through the venous system in search of another male with which she can again mate. Figure 11.7 shows a diagrammatic impression of the life cycle.

Clinical course
In the human there are 3 stages of the disease.

Stage of invasion or allergic stage
This occurs 3 or 4 days after invasion by the host and is characterised by an irritation of the skin which encourages scratching but which soon passes off. In many cases the symptoms are trivial and are completely ignored.

Stage of generalisation or febrile stage
This comes on 4 to 6 weeks after the initial infestation. The patients experience fever, lassitude and fatigue, which slowly passes off, and is due to the migration of the worm from the liver to the pelvic organs.

Stage of localisation
This is related to the time when the worms have reached the target organ, usually the ureter and the bladder, and it is during this stage, that the patients may complain of haematuria, frequency and dysuria.

Treatment
The traditional treatment is antimony tartrate, given as tartar emetic by the intravenous route, 2 ml of a 6 per cent solution every other day for 15 injections. Although highly effective, the therapeutic potential is limited by its toxicity, which governs the dosage of the drug, which can be given, with safety. Relapses, therefore, occur but repeated courses can be given at 6 month intervals. The antimony compounds exert their effect on the ovum and miracadia as well as the adult worms.

Within the last decade a new drug ambilhar has been introduced. This has the merit of being given by the oral route as well as being reliable, simple and safe. It is given in a dose of 25 mg/kilo of body weight, in two equally divided doses for 7 days. The most important side effect, is a reaction in the central nervous system, but this can be effectively reduced by administering either barbiturate or diazepan with the ambilhar. Ambilhar stains the urine brown. This is not significant, but it serves as a reliable indication that the patient is taking the drug.

The relative place of these two drugs in the treatment of bilharzia has not been finally resolved, and many authorities still feel that tartar emetic gives the best results. However, there is no doubt that a high proportion of patients can be cured of the initial infection, but the problem of continuous reinfection remains, and until this aspect has been overcome, the eradication of the disease remains a formidable challenge.

Localisation of the disease
It must be appreciated that bilharzia is a venous disease, and that the organs likely to be affected are those which have a rich venous supply. Two important areas are at L.3 where there is a large plexus of veins due to anastomosis between branches from the lumbar veins, inferior mesenteric veins, the left spermatic vein and the left periureteric veins. The second area, is at the lower end of the left ureter, where there is another large plexus formed from branches of the inferior

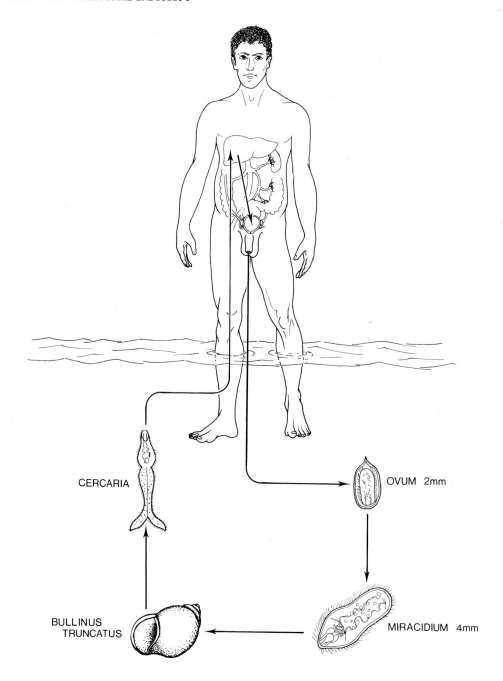

Fig. 11.7   Diagrammatic representation of the life cycle of the worm schistosoma haematobium.

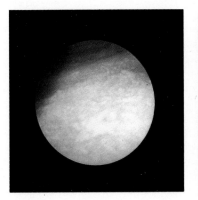

Fig. 11.8
Bilharzia cystitis cystica.

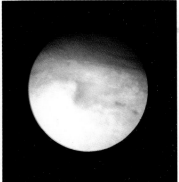

Fig. 11.9
Cystitis granularis. Note atrophic
mucous membrane.

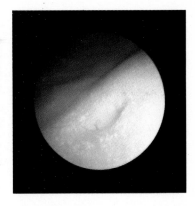

Fig. 11.10
Sandy patch close to ureteric
orifice.

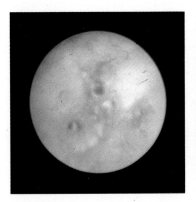

Fig. 11.11
Dead bilharzia ova.

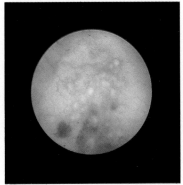

Fig. 11.12
Active bilharzia with ova about to
cross mucous membrane.

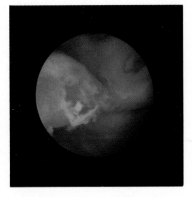

Fig. 11.13
Bilharzia ulcer superimposed on
bladder neck sclerosis.

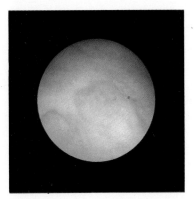

Fig. 11.14
Hypertrophic sessile polyp with
sandy area.

mesenteric vein, the superior and inferior vesical veins and the superior haemorrhoidal vein.

Pathological progress

The initial pathology occurs in the submucosa and the subsequent changes can either be atrophic or hypertrophic, depending on the reaction of the mucous membrane to the ovum. The final pathological state can be either healing, which is rare, or one of the many other states, e.g. proliperation, ulceration, fibrosis, stenosis, fistulae formation, calcification or neoplastic changes.

Areas of bladder affected

As bilharzia is a disease affecting venous channels, the areas of the bladder affected, are those, where the venous sinuses are most concentrated in the submucous tissue. Lesions are, therefore, usually seen in the posterolateral aspects of the bladder, close to the left ureteric orifice and just above the trigone. The trigone is rarely involved, as, not only, is there hardly any submucous layer, but also it is the area of the bladder that moves the least, so that ova are hardly ever deposited.

Bladder changes

The bladder changes can affect the mucosa, submucosa, muscle and perivesical tissues.

Mucosa

These changes can either be acute or chronic. If acute, they are seen as a patchy cystitis or an acute granulomatous cystitis, which is difficult to distinguish from a simple non-specific cystitis. If the lesion becomes chronic, the mucosa becomes dull or can progress to cystitis cystica or cystitis granuloma. Cystitis cystica (Fig. 11.8), is caused by a hypertrophic reaction of the mucous membrane, which enfolds itself and coalesces with another similar fold to form an enclosed space, and which then secretes mucous, forming a cyst. Cystitis granulosis (Fig. 11.9), is caused by the same hypertrophic folds of mucous membrane joining with other folds to form a solid stricture. Both these changes are permanent, though they may vary in degree. They are the result of the disease and not indicative of an active process. At this stage of the disease, the mucous is pale and atrophic and is clearly seen in this photograph.

Submubosa

The changes that are most often seen are sandy patches (Fig. 11.10), which are formed by atrophy of the mucous membrane, which loses its pink vascular appearance and becomes dull and anaemic and covers old calcified bilharzia ova, which are buried immediately beneath the surface. Such areas are an indication, not of active disease, but of old healed lesions. They are permanent, a relic of past infection. Tubercles (Fig. 11.11) may also be seen. They appear as seed-like yellowish bodies, 1–2 mm in diameter, which may look shiny and vesicular, almost transparent. Alternatively, they may appear as a light brown promitary, surrounded by inflammation (Fig. 11.12), which is an indication of an active process. Superficial ulcers (Fig. 11.13), may also be seen. They are small, irregular, pale with a definitive margin, and a yellowish base. They may be simple or multiple and can be seen superimposed in sclerotic areas, particularly at the bladder neck (Fig. 11.13). Such ulcers are evidence of an acute disease. They can heal with treatment, leaving a thin stellate scar. Another change that can be seen in the bladder, is the bilharzia papilloma (Fig. 11.14). These are caused by an infection of the submucosa by ova, which cause the mucosa to protrude and form polypoidal swellings. They are sessile, have no fronds, are immobile, stunted and darker in colour. Some undergo malignant changes, and occasionally, the centre of the sessile papilloma, may slough forming a bilharzia ulcer.

Muscle

Once the muscle has become involved, the bladder becomes irritated and the capacity steadily decreases, due to fibrosis and calcification. When this state has been reached, frequency of micturition becomes intolerable, so that an enterocystoplasty has to be carried out.

Perivesical tissue

When the disease has developed to this extent a mass can be felt on bimanual examination and an intravenous urogram shows a distorted bladder. Invariably, in this type of case, both ureters will have become involved and will have stenosed at the ureterovesical junction causing dilatation and calcification, followed by hydronephrosis and a deteriorating kidney function. Such extensive disease is not uncommon in areas where the disease is endemic, and not only poses problems, which tax the ingenuity of urologists experienced in its treatment, but also may present in a manner, which is beyond surgical treatment due to irreparable renal damage, causing irreversible renal failure.

REFERENCES

Badenoch, A. W. (1971). Chronic interstitial cystitis. *British Journal of Urology*, **43**, 718.

Editorial, British Medical Journal. Interstitial cystitis. *British Medical Journal*, **1**, 644.

Ellis, H. (1969). *A History of Bladder Stones*. Blackwell Scientific Publications, Oxford & Edinburgh.

Makar, Naguib. *Urological Aspects of Bilharziasis in Egypt*. S.O.P. Press, Cairo, 1955.

12. Bladder tumours

Bladder tumours take up a large part of a urologist's time. They are a serious condition, and one, which is not always easily accepted by the patients, as the treatment may be unpleasant and the subsequent supervision prolonged. It is essential, therefore, that there should be early mutual confidence between the urologist and the patient, if the best results are to be achieved. Ninety per cent of bladder tumours arise in the transitional epithelium of the bladder wall, and the remainder form a miscellaneous rare group. They are uncommon before the age of 30, and the great majority occur at the ages between 60 and 80 years. About 2 per cent of all deaths, from malignancy, are attributed to bladder tumours. Males are affected more than females in the ratio of 3 : 1. The cause, as with all forms of malignancy, is largely unknown. However, there are some recognised carcinogens, which may precipitate bladder tumour formation, notably beta-naphthylamine and benzidrine. They also occur after schistosomiasis infection of the bladder, but in this condition, the pathology is usually squamous epithelium of high malignancy. In all cases of bladder tumours, a careful examination of the kidney and ureters is essential, as conincidental tumours, in these areas, do occur. The common presenting symptom is haematuria, and it is a symptom which should never be underestimated or ignored. Once a patient presents with such a symptom, however brief the attack, either macroscopic or microscopic, it should be fully investigated. Most patients will approach their doctor after an attack of haematuria, but it is not uncommon to find some who have had three or even more attacks, going back over a period of a year or longer. This is unfortunate, as the longer the patient delays seeking medical advice from the onset of haematuria, the worse are the results of treatment. Physical examination rarely gives any vital information, but occasionally extensive tumours may be palpated in the region of the fundus of the bladder, or even invading the paravesical tissues. In these types of tumour, the lesions are usually far beyond surgical treatment.

Investigations

Intravenous pyelography

This examination should be carried out using a high dose technique, preferably incorporating a dynamic study, using the image intensifier. In this way, the dye can be seen passing down the ureter, and small filling defects in the ureter, which otherwise might be missed, may be seen. Usually, the radiographic appearance of the bladder is normal, but if the lesion is extensive, some irregularity of the wall or a filling defect, may be noticed.

Urine cystology

Urine cytology is unlikely to give much information in the initial examination of a new case, and is probably unnecessary. It is, however, important in those patients, who are attending for follow-up examinations, and who, for one reason or another, present a distinct hazard to the anaesthetist. It can be used as a screen and if there are any suspected cells, cystoscopy should then be carried out, if necessary, under local anaesthesia. Johnson, in 1964, stated that urine cytology should be accurate in 90 per cent of cases.

Cystourethroscopy

Cystourethroscopy is the essential investigation. The urethroscopy should be carried out first, and should be followed, immediately, by a careful examination of the whole of the bladder. Both these investigations ought to be performed under general anaesthesia, and if any tumours or suspicious areas are seen, a biopsy must be taken. In addition, a careful examination of the whole of the mucous membrane of the bladder, between the tumours is made, and further biopsies taken to exclude carcinoma *in situ*. Areas of inflammation, distant from tumours, are particularly suspect, and a separate biopsy of these areas should always be performed. Both ureteric orifices are carefully watched until more than one efflux is seen from each side, because, if there is a co-existing tumour in the ureter, a haemorrhagic efflux may be seen. In addition, small tumours in the intramural part of the ureter can appear at the orifice, when an efflux is taking place. At the same time as this examination, a bimanual examination of the bladder is performed with a finger in the rectum or the vagina and the hand on the hypogastrium, the bladder being palpated between the two hands. This is an important examination, but its limitations should be realised. In the first place, small tumours cannot be felt; secondly, if the patient is obese, examination is difficult and can be misleading, as it is almost impossible to achieve an accurate feel of the tumour, especially when it is soft with limited invasion of the bladder wall. However, it is this examination, on which the T grading is partly made, so it must always be performed. But, it cannot be too strongly stressed, that a biopsy of all tumours and especially the area surrounding the base should be taken, so that the T grading can be confirmed by the histopathological examination. It is the histopathological examination that largely governs the assessment of the best method of treatment.

Classification of tumours

The classification of tumours which has been accepted is the TNM classification of the UICC published in 1974 and this appears at the end of this chapter. The most important part of this classification is the 'T' element, which is essential for accurate prognosis, and Figure 12.1 shows the meaning of this classification. The pictures that follow are based on this classification and it was felt that the value of the endoscopic appearance would be increased if the histopathological picture of the bladder photograph were mounted alongside. Figures 12.2 and 12.3 show the microscopic appearance of a carcinoma *in situ*, which is described as definite anaplasia of surface epithelium where the formation of papillary structures are without infiltration. These are lesions, which assimilate carcinoma, but which show, initially, very little invasion. They are usually seen close to an existing tumour, but also may appear elsewhere in the bladder, and many patients are first diagnosed by cytological examination. If the condition is suspected, then a good practice is to take biopsy

specimens from six or seven areas in the bladder thus covering as wide an area as possible. These tumours in the early stages may not be visible by the endoscope, but if there are changes in the mucous membrane, endoscopic resection is the treatment of choice. It is important that the bladder be examined frequently over a considerable length of time, starting at three-monthly intervals and when there has been no recurrence for two to three years, gradually extending the intervals for examination to once a year. This is necessary as, in about 30 per cent of these cases an invasive carcinoma occurs. This condition may be symptomless, but it can be mistaken for a recurrent urinary tract infection. Males are more commonly infected than females and haematuria is invariably present, although often microscopic. If the recurrence rate is rapid, it is impossible to be certain that the lesion has been completely excised by endoscopic techniques or that other tumours may not appear in different parts of the bladder. In these cases of recurrence, it is prudent to give a course of irradiation to the whole of the bladder. However, when the invasion of tissues has commenced, it is doubtful whether endoscopic surgery and radiatherapy will be successful, and cystectomy is then the only alternative. Figures 12.4, 12.5 and 12.6 show a papillary differentiated T1 tumour with the histological picture of a papillary intermediate carcinoma. These are often small lesions, and it can be appreciated how difficult and almost impossible it is for these tumours to be felt by bimanual examination. The tumours may be single or multiple; they can be large, 5 g or more, in which case they can be felt as a soft swelling inside the bladder (Figs. 12.7 & 12.8). Once diagnosed, they should be resected as soon as possible. They are always limited to the superficial layers of the bladder and do not penetrate beyond the *lamina propria*. Occasionally, the tumours are of a more solid nature and indicate intermediate malignancy. Figures 12.9 and 12.10 show a solid intermediate transisitional cell carcinoma invading the *lamina propria*. It is essential to ensure that in all these tumours, the excision goes beyond what appears to be the margin of the tumour or the stalk and the mucous membrane should be excised for at least 2 cm around the tumour, including the superficial muscle. Figure 12.11 shows the appearance of the bladder after resection, and the muscle fibres can be clearly seen. Even if, it is felt, that a complete excision has taken place, repeated endoscopic examinations should be arranged, as the recurrence rate is approximately 40 per cent of cases. Figure 12.12 shows a recurrence close to an original tumour, which appears as a white scarred area. However, if there is no recurrence in five years, it is reasonable as a screening procedure, that urinary cytology should be carried out on a yearly basis. If the tumour were found to be multiple, at the initial

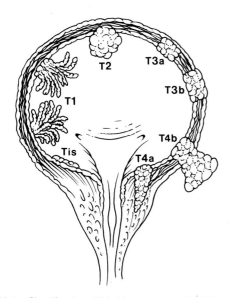

Fig. 12.1 Classification of bladder tumours—the 'T' elements.

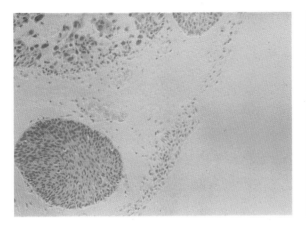

Fig. 12.2
Histological picture of carcinoma *in situ* in Von Brunns rest.

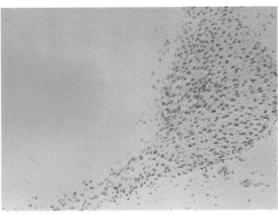

Fig. 12.3
Histological picture of focal *in situ* carcinoma.

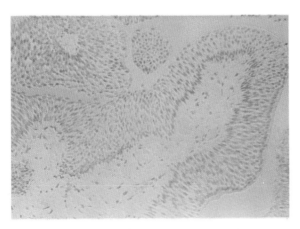

Fig. 12.4
T1 carcinoma.

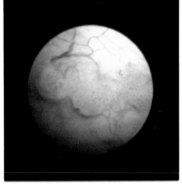

Fig. 12.5
Papillary differentiated transitional cell carcinoma with intact basement membrane.

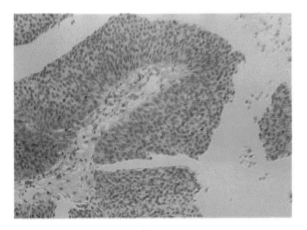

Fig. 12.6
Papillary differentiated transitional cell carcinoma with basement membrane breakthrough.

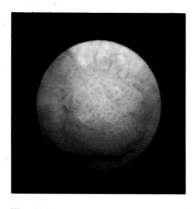

Fig. 12.7
Papillary intermediate T1 carcinoma.

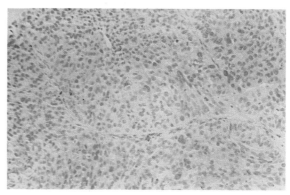

Fig. 12.8
Histology of papillary intermediate carcinoma.

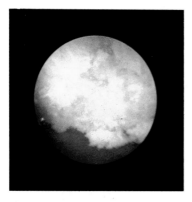

Fig. 12.9
Solid intermediate transitional cell
carcinoma invading the *lamina propria*.

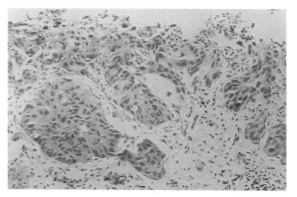

Fig. 12.10
Histology of solid transitional cell carcinoma invading the
lamina propria.

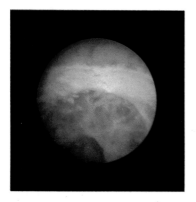

Fig. 12.11
Appearance of the bladder after
excision of an early carcinoma showing
honeycomb appearance of muscle fibres.

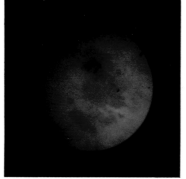

Fig. 12.12
Recurrent carcinoma close to site of
original excision.

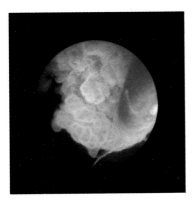

Fig. 12.13
Bladder carcinoma before being treated
by Helmstein's procedure.

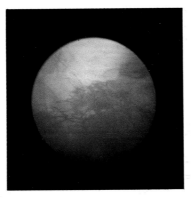

Fig. 12.14
Bladder carcinoma after being treated
by Helmstein's procedure.

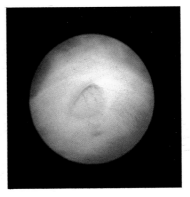

Fig. 12.15
Ureteric orifice in centre of scar
tissue.

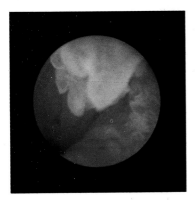

Fig. 12.16
Papillary and solid T2 carcinoma
invading muscle.

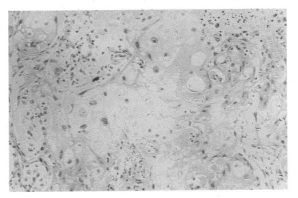

Fig. 12.17
Histology of solid T2 anaplastic carcinoma invading muscle.

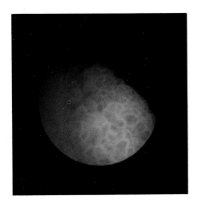

Fig. 12.18
Solid T3 carcinoma.

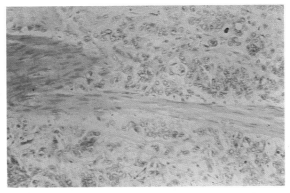

Fig. 12.19
Histology of solid T3 carcinoma through muscle.

examination, it is suggested that there is some change in the normal epithelium, which indicates that it is likely that the tumour will recur, from time to time, in different parts of the bladder. About 90 per cent of such tumours can be kept under control by endoscopic surgery, provided that it is frequent and complete. However, if the multiple tumours are too numerous to be controlled by endoscopic diathermy, some other method of treatment will be necessary. These multiple superficial tumours can be treated and kept under control by Epodyl 100 ml of 1 per cent solution instilled into the bladder. The patient should be encouraged to hold it in the bladder for as long as possible. This treatment is continued daily for ten days and then weekly for three months. Forty per cent of patients do not respond to this method of treatment for any length of time, and once further recurrence of the tumour has occurred, cystectomy and urinary diversion become inevitable, as the spread through the bladder can be rapid. Endoscopic resection should not be used once Epodyl has failed to control the tumour, as it can never be certain that all the recurrent lesions have been eradicated. Occasionally, bladder tumours are extensive, some weighing over 100 g, and appear to cover the whole of the bladder mucous membrane. Many of these tumours are of low grade malignancy, and in these cases, Helmstein's procedure as an initial treatment may help to reduce the bulk of the tumour, so that it can then be treated by endoscopic resection. The bladder is kept distended under epidural anaesthesia, for four or five hours by means of an indwelling catheter, and this destroys the large part of the superficial tumour formation. It is possible at the end of three or four weeks to excise this residual tumour by endoscopic resection. Figures 12.13 and 12.14 show the picture of such a carcinoma of the bladder before and after being treated by Helmstein's procedure. T1 tumours may also occur at the ureteric orifice. These are particularly difficult to treat, as it is never possible to be certain that the resection or treatment by diathermy coagulation will completely destroy the tumour. Furthermore, it is impossible to say that there is no other tumour formation 2 or 3 cm up the ureter. If, after the initial resection, the tumour returns, then this tumour should be excised together with the lower 3″ of ureter and a cuff of the bladder, containing the ureteric orifice, with reimplantation of the ureter using a reflux-preventing technique. This procedure should only be carried out, if it is reasonably certain that there are no other tumours in the proximal part of the ureter. Tumours may surround a ureteric orifice, so that it becomes invisible. In these cases, the ureteric orifice should be ignored and the tumour completely resected. Stenosis of the ureter is rare, but reflux more common, as at the time of the first follow-up examination the orifice is re-epithelialised

and appears in the centre of an area of scar tissue (Fig. 12.15). Occasionally, when there are small multiple or superficial tumours irradiation can be used. Although most of the tumours are insensitive to irradiation, nevertheless, some excellent results can be achieved. Extensive irradiation to the bladder, 5 or 6000 rads can produce quite a severe and intensive irradiation cystitis, which causes patchy areas of inflammation giving rise to haematuria and frequency of micturition. The bladder changes usually heal spontaneously in two or three months, but occasionally, the irradiation causes intramural fibrosis and a small contracted bladder. If haematuria is also a recurring problem in this type of case, it rarely stops spontaneously, and cystectomy may be necessary to control the haemorrhage.

Invasive bladder tumours

T2 and T3

Endoscopic resection is now generally accepted as the first method of treatment for T1 lesions. There is still considerable debate as to the best method of treatment of the T2 and T3 groups. With regard to the T2, where there is limited infiltration satisfactory results can be obtained by endoscopic surgery. Figures 12.16 and 12.17 show a papillary solid T2 carcinoma invading muscle. Once the lesion has reached T3, then endoscopic resection is almost completely inadequate, and Figures 12.18 and 12.19 show a T3 lesion which has invaded muscle. The resection, in many cases, has almost completely gone through the bladder muscle and further resection would not be possible without the risk of perforation of the bladder. In these cases, there are three courses of action from which to choose. Firstly, endoscopic resection of as much of the tumour as possible, followed by irradiation either by high voltage X-ray or cobalt beam. Secondly, excision of the tumour through a transvesical approach and implantation, of either gold or radon seeds, into the tumour and surrounding mucous membrane. Thirdly, cystectomy and diversion. In all these cases, frequent follow-up cystoscopic examinations must be carried out, as recurrences are almost inevitable. It is probable that extensive endoscopic resection followed by high-dosage irradiation will give as good a result from the survival point of view, as opening the bladder and inserting gold or radon seeds. Furthermore, such a method of treatment obviates the necessity of open surgery. However, it can only be emphasised that the results of T2 and T3 lesions are very poor and the cure rate is low. All the surgeon can do is to carry out palliative procedures in the hope that there will be some symptomatic improvement, but it is very doubtful whether it could alter the ultimate course of the disease, except in the cases of a few patients.

T4 lesions

The prognosis of T4 lesions is grave indeed, and very few survive more than a year after commencing treatment, and in these cases, surgery has nothing to offer. Radiotherapy can be introduced as a palliative procedure. It gives some symptomatic improvement in a few cases. The main function of the physician in treating these patients, in whom the disease has reached this extent, is to treat symptoms and keep the patient as free from pain as possible. Chemotherapy has been used, but the results are poor; furthermore toxic effects were frequent, including aggranulocytosis. Cystectomy has been performed in some cases, but in many, on exploration, the tumour is found to be so fixed that excision is impossible. There may also be glands along the aorta and even secondaries in the liver. Palliative urinary diversion has been suggested by some authors, but it is very doubtful whether it is justified, as the management only presents another problem for the patient.

CLASSIFICATION OF TUMOURS

The meaning of the TNM symbols are as follows:

T—clinical examination, urography, cystoscopy, bimanual examination under full anaesthesia and biopsy or transurethral resection of the tumour if indicated prior to definitive treatment.

N—clinical examination, lymphography and urography.

M—clinical examination, chest X-ray and biochemical tests and the more advanced primary tumours or when clinical suspicion warrants, radiographic isotope studies should be done.

Classification as applied to bladder tumours

T—primary tumour.

Tls—Preinvasive carcinoma, carcinoma *in situ*.

Tx—the minimal requirements to assess fully the extent of the primary tumour cannot be met.

To—no evidence of primary tumour.

T1—On bimanual examination a freely mobile mass may be felt. This should not be felt after complete transurethral resection of the lesion and/or microscopically the tumour does not extend beyond the *lamina propria*.

T2—bimanual examination, there is induration of the bladder wall which is mobile. There is no residual induration after complete transurethral resection of the lesion and/or there is microscopic invasion of superficial muscle.

T3—on bimanual examination induration or a nodular mobile mass is palpable in the bladder wall, which persists after transurethral resection of the resection of the exophytic part of the lesion and/or there is microscopic invasion of deep muscle or of extension through the bladder wall.

T3a—invasion of deep muscle.

T3b—extension through the bladder wall.

T4—tumour fixed or invading neighbouring structures and/or there is microscopic evidence of such an involvement.

T4a—tumour invading prostate, uterus or vagina.

T4b—tumour fixed to the pelvic wall and/or infiltrating the abdominal wall.

Histo-pathological categories

P—an assessment of the P categories is based on evidence derived from surgical operation and histopathology, i.e. when a tissue other than biopsy is available for examination. The suffix M may be added to the appropriate P category to indicate multiple tumours, e.g. P2M.

Pls—preinvasive carcinoma, carcinoma *in situ*.

Px—the extent of invasion cannot be assessed.

Po—no tumour found on examination of specimen.

P1—tumour not extending beyond the *lamina propria*.

P2—tumour with infiltration of superficial muscle not more than half way through the muscle coat.

P3—tumour with infiltration of deep muscle more than half way through the muscle coat or infiltration of perivesical tissue.

P4—tumour with infiltration of prostate or other extra vesical strictures.

G—histopathological grading

Gx—grade cannot be assessed.

Go—no evidence of anaplasia, i.e. papilloma.

G1—low grade malignancy.

G2—medium grade malignancy.

G3—high grade malignancy.

Index